PATIENT CARE

Patient Care

Death and Life in the Emergency Room

Paul Seward, MD

Catapult 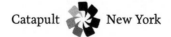 New York

Some names and identifying details have been changed
to protect the privacy of individuals.

To my teachers, who gave me their knowledge

To my mentors, who gave me their wisdom

To my patients, who gave me their trust

To Linda, who has given me everything

Contents

Preface

M Y GOAL IN writing this book is to tell the reader what it's like to work in the emergency room. I don't mean just what happens there; rather I mean what it feels like to work there.

It is true that feelings arise in response to things that happen. Therefore, a book about experiences must also be a book of stories. Even so, as much as possible, the stories in this book are about situations, not merely events. An event is just something that happens; a situation is something that, as it happens, asks for a response from the people who are witnesses.

In light of that distinction, it is important that you, the reader, know that, as much as possible, these stories are true. If they differ from what someone else remembers, that is due to three things: time, perspective, and privacy.

First, these stories occurred during a professional life of well over forty years, in a practice that took me to hospitals in California, Washington, and Arizona on the West Coast, to Georgia in the South, and to New York on the East Coast. I could not possibly remember all the details of those occasions, or the conversations I had. Nonetheless, the core truths of these stories are written from memories that I could not forget if I tried. So if I have fleshed out some details, or put some of my own words in people's mouths, I have done so not to change the truth of the events but simply to make those truths accessible.

Second, everyone sees from where they stand. Others who were present are assuredly entitled to have differences in what they experienced and remember. However, the only memories I can give you are my own. Those I have rendered as honestly as I can.

Finally, where I could do so, I have made changes that do not alter the meaning of the situation but honor the privacy of the patients and family members who were involved. These are things such as people's ages, or gender; or the city or time in which the situations took place. Also, I have seen cases like the ones I have chosen many, many times. Thus, if you think that you recognize any particular patient, rest assured, you don't.

With those disclaimers, everything I have put here actually did happen, and for better or worse, I was there in the role I have described. If I have done my job, then what you see is what I saw and what I remember.

However, I have a second goal as well. For me, part of the reason I worked in the ER was that I found it to be a place where I was asked to do the work of living. There was a question on my medical school application: "Why do you want to be a doctor?" My answer was that, in my opinion, being a doctor was the best way I could think of to do two things:

first to study, in depth and in detail, just what a human being really is; and then to act on the implications of what I had learned.

That answer seems pretentious to me now. I was only twenty then, and now, in my seventies, I have seen very clearly that all walks of life offer that challenge and that opportunity. But at that age, I saw it most clearly in medicine. So I went to medical school. And a half century later, I have indeed acquired a few beliefs about the question of who we are and what we should be doing.

The one that is relevant to this book is very simple: I believe that the principal reason we are on this planet is to have our noses constantly rubbed in our obligation to care about people who are strangers to us. When I look around, I see a world in which, in every instant of our lives, we are unavoidably confronted with the question of whether the quality of other people's lives and experiences is as important as our own. If we think so, we will act in one way; if we do not, then we will act in another.

But why is caring about strangers so difficult? Are we not hardwired for love? We naturally love our children and our family, we care about our friends. Of course we do. For almost all of human history, those were the only people we ever encountered. We had to love them to survive.

Yet I would argue that precisely because those behaviors are so hardwired, they are not matters of choice. Love, as a choice, enters the picture only when we encounter a stranger. Our instinct to care for our family and our tribe does not extend to them. That kind of caring must be learned. And, in my opinion, the ER is a place that, if you are paying any attention at all, will teach you that lesson.

But—and this is the final and most critical point—the belief that we are here to learn to love others not only motivates such choices, it is created by them. Yes, certain environments teach some values better than others. But like any other school, the most important part of learning is the desire of the pupil to become better than they already are.

For much of my life, I have tried my best to enact the role of a caring physician. I have no idea whether I have succeeded at all in becoming one, but I do know what it felt like to try.

PATIENT CARE

CHAPTER ONE

The Young Man's Friend

I T WAS MIDAFTERNOON. As I recall, it was not a particularly busy one.

The chart was not the next one in the rack; it never even got to the rack. Instead, while I was writing a note about a patient whose hand laceration I had just closed, the nurse covering the back hall came up front to the main nurses' station where I was working. She didn't say anything. She just stood there waiting silently, arms folded over her chest, holding a chart within them.

I finished the sentence I was writing and looked up. "What do you need?" I asked.

"I wonder if you could come and see this one now. He's pretty sick." I stood up at once.

I knew that his being sick wasn't the only reason she had come to the front. After all, this was an emergency room. Most people were sick, or at least thought they were. Furthermore, patients who were critically unstable went to the resuscitation rooms, not to the back hall. But if she had wanted to say more at that point, she would have done so. I just said "Okay," took the chart, and followed her.

On the way, I looked over what was written: a twenty-two-year-old man, resident of a nursing home; normally in a chronic vegetative state; noted this morning to have a fever and be less responsive than his baseline level, which wasn't much to start with. His vital signs (pulse, respiratory rate, blood pressure, and temperature are together called that because that is exactly what they are—vital) showed a blood pressure of 125/60, a heart rate of 120, a respiratory rate of 20, and a rectal temperature of 103.5. I walked a little faster.

Fever, rapid heart and respiratory rate, and diminished activity.

He probably just had the flu. But as I often told the residents, we aren't in the "probably" business; our business is "Let's make sure."

At the same time, what struck me the most was the patient's age: why was a twenty-two-year-old man vegetating in a nursing home?

The nurse was walking beside me now. "Do we have an old chart on this guy?" I asked.

"I got it already. It's in the room." She had been an ER nurse for a while. I had learned very early that if you allow nurses to keep you from making terrible mistakes, they will be happy to do so. They just need to know that it isn't a dangerous thing to do.

Okay, I thought. Let's take a look.

At first glance, the patient looked like a normal young man, lying on his back, asleep, with his head raised on a pillow. However, at second glance he didn't look normal at all.

From across the room, it was apparent that he was breathing rapidly—twenty breaths per minute or so—but also with the noisy snoring respirations of someone who wasn't controlling his airway very well. Therefore, the first thing we did was crank up the head of his bed a little more, adjust his pillow, and pull his jaw slightly forward. His breathing eased at once, but he did not awaken and his respirations remained rapid. He was also slightly pale, with dry skin that was warm to the touch and without an obvious rash. When I listened to his chest, I could hear good breath sounds on both sides but I could also hear fluid in his bronchial passages and possibly in his lungs as well. His abdomen was soft, but there were none of the occasional quiet gurgling noises that healthy bowels make.

Most important, he gave no sign that he was aware of us. When I pinched the skin above his shoulder and rubbed my knuckle on his chest, he made vague movements with his hands but no real attempt to stop me or push me away.

He was obviously ill with some generalized infection—whether in his blood, lungs, nervous system, urinary tract, or even bowel, I didn't know. But his unresponsiveness was out of proportion to a simple infection—even a serious one.

And of course, there was the matter of the "chronic vegetative state." Was his unresponsiveness just how he was, or was the infection contributing to it?

At this moment, such distinctions didn't matter. One rule of emergency medicine is that when you aren't sure what is going on, first take care of the patient; then let the diagnosis emerge. The first thing we needed to do was to protect his life. Only after that might we have the luxury of trying to figure out all the things that were wrong with him.

He was certainly both infected and dehydrated, so I asked the nurse to draw blood for laboratory evaluation—the tray was already in the room—and to start a large-bore IV, an intravenous line that uses a needle with a large diameter in order to permit rapid flow. Then she should run in a liter of normal saline as fast as it would go. He would also need a Foley catheter to measure urine flow and obtain a sterile specimen, then a chest X-ray and a separate set of blood cultures. Finally, after the blood cultures were drawn, but still as quickly as possible, we needed to give him some broad-spectrum antibiotics.

I started to add that we should move him to a room better suited for resuscitation and get ready to intubate him. But then I stopped. His airway was now good and his vital signs were stable—at least for the moment. His oxygen saturation was good. Furthermore, we could do everything we needed to do immediately, right where he was. Also, I wanted to think about him for just a moment, before I made any big decisions.

"On it," the nurse said. Then, pointing at the thick manila folder on the counter, she said, "There's a discharge summary from his last admission." Then she started working on the IV.

I picked up the chart, pulled out the three-page typewritten summary that was just inside the front cover, and read through it rapidly.

He hadn't always been in a nursing home. Until he was nineteen, he had been a normal young man; normal, that is, if "normal" includes getting into trouble in high school, experimenting with drugs, and running with a hard crowd. He had also had a girlfriend and evidently cared about her. She had gotten pregnant, and although he hadn't married her, he had stayed with her and worked a couple of jobs to care for her and their son.

Unfortunately, it turned out that one part of his earnings came from selling drugs. And one night, about two years prior, things had gone badly. There had been an argument— about money? About the drugs? The author of the note did not seem to know. What was clear, however, was that during that argument, the young man had been struck hard over the head with an iron pipe, fracturing his skull and causing a massive contusion of his brain. He had been taken to the ER and then admitted to the neurosurgical service, where he had had immediate surgery to drain blood from around his brain. They had even temporarily removed the top of his skull so that the swelling of the brain would not cause increased pressure. They treated his seizures with anticonvulsant medication, made sure he had adequate oxygen and glucose, and put him in a barbiturate-induced coma to see whether things would settle down and recover on their own. In short, excellent intensive neurosurgical care saved his life.

Sort of. The only thing they were unable to do was wake him up.

So since that time he had lain in bed in a nursing home. He had a tube that went through the abdominal wall directly into his stomach and through which he was fed. He was turned regularly and had his diaper changed as often as necessary. His eyes were frequently open, but he did not look particularly at faces; nor did he respond to any speech or say anything himself. His mother visited him frequently and she thought that at times he recognized her. The nurses were doubtful.

He had been to our hospital several times over the last couple of years. Once he had been brought in because the tube into his stomach had fallen out and needed to be replaced. A couple of other times he was brought in for respiratory and urinary tract infections. But this was the first time he had been this sick.

I read all this. And then I looked him over once more. And then I looked up at the nurse.

"Listen," I said. "Can you draw everything—but then hold the tubes here—don't send them. Then, when you have his IV started and have given him his fluid bolus, set the IV at twenty cc's per hour and come tell me how he's doing. I have to make a phone call."

Let's pause for a moment. At that point in his care, I realized that this young man was more than just a problem with an infection. I needed to think about how to care for him as a human being. Given his situation, what might he really need from us? And how could we possibly discover what that was?

Certainly his presentation posed some important medical questions—about infection, about the recognition and management of early septic shock, even about managing breathing in a patient who has a badly damaged nervous system and trouble maintaining his blood pressure.

But humans have more than medical problems. What about ethical questions? Quality-of-life questions? What about spiritual or religious questions? And who should be involved in both asking and answering these questions, for clearly the patient could no longer do so?

Equally important, I was not meeting him as a pastor of a parishioner in church, or as a teacher of a student in school. He had presented to me as a patient in an emergency room and I was there as the physician tasked to provide his emergency care. That setting and those roles all by themselves exert a powerful demand to provide, without hesitation, a highly technical and expert form of care, to do everything possible to save his life, to cure his injury. That was my role. But as a human being, confronted with the needs of another human being, to what extent was it my job to simply enact that role, and to what extent was it my duty to look beyond it?

Let me say up front that, over thirty years later, I do not pretend to know the answers. But even then, I knew that not knowing the answers did not excuse me from having to provide them. Whether or not I wanted to be, I was the person who had the knowledge and the authority to act on his behalf. Whatever I did for this young man—or refrained from doing—was a responsibility that I could not avoid. I had chosen to be here—had worked and studied for many years to be here. I had been hired by the hospital and was paid well to be in precisely this position, to make these decisions—and to choose correctly.

So what did I choose to do?

I sat down at the dictation station that I had left a few minutes before, picked up the phone, and dialed the number that was listed on the front page of the chart. After only one ring, a woman answered. I gave my name and asked for hers. Then I said that I was calling from the hospital and that I was the emergency physician caring for her son.

I don't remember the details of our conversation. The gist of it was that she had already been called by the nursing home and had been expecting my call. She asked how he was doing. I said that he was very sick, that he plainly had a serious infection—his lung examination indicated that it was probably pneumonia—from which, given his underlying problems, he could very easily die. I also said that I had given him some fluids and that, for the moment, he was stable, but if we were to save his life, we would need to do much more and very soon. I asked if she had any feelings about that, one way or the other. She said that she could be there in a few minutes and could I wait until she arrived? I said that we would hold off till then and hung up the phone. I asked the ward clerk to page both the patient representative (a person hired by a hospital who makes phone calls, finds magazines, brings coffee, and generally makes sure that patients and their families are cared about as well as cared for) and the hospital chaplain, then went back to the young man's room to see how he was doing.

His mother arrived in under fifteen minutes. The patient representative had been watching for her, had met her in the waiting room, and brought her back to be with her son. I was still in the room, and when his mother entered, she went directly to his side, took his hand, and looked carefully into his face. She spoke to him then, telling him that she was here and that she loved him. Then she looked up at me.

I asked the nurse if she could stay with the patient for a couple of minutes. Then the patient rep and I took the mother to a small room nearby, meant for families of seriously ill patients, to wait in privacy. It had a real carpet on the floor, as well as a couch and a couple of chairs, and end tables furnished with lamps and magazines.

Our conversation did not take long. She asked how her son was. I said that for the moment, with fluids, his heart rate and blood pressure had improved slightly. We had given him a Tylenol suppository, which had had a minimal effect on his fever, and that might have made him more comfortable, even if he could not let us know.

Next, she asked what was going to happen. I said that on the one hand, if we gave him a mixture of strong antibiotics and admitted him to the critical care unit for intensive care, it was possible that he would live to return to the nursing home. On the other hand, without antibiotics I felt that he would probably die within a few hours. I also said that as far as we could tell, there was no indication that he was suffering any pain.

Then I told her that I could not say whether it was better to try to save his life for now, knowing that this episode would surely be followed by more of the same, or to let him go in peace. That was a decision that only she could make.

His mother was silent for a moment. Then she said, "I think we need to let him go." I nodded and got up to help her back to the room.

At that moment, the chaplain tapped on the door, put in his head, and asked if he could join us. He was a quiet man, humorous when humor was needed, calm and caring always. He did not wear clerical garb, just khaki pants, a dress shirt and tie, and a name tag identifying him simply as "Chaplain."

He was Christian—Baptist, I think—but he cared for everyone in the same way, meeting them within their beliefs without pressing his own.

I introduced him to the patient's mother and asked her whether I could tell him what was going on. She nodded, and I gave him a brief outline of the situation and what the mother had decided. Then the three of us walked back to the patient's room. The patient rep had gone to get the mother some coffee and around that time returned. She gave her the cup and, without asking any questions, went with us. The mother and the chaplain then went inside.

I stayed outside for a moment and told the nurse and the patient rep the plan, and asked if they were okay with being a part of what was happening. They both nodded, and so the three of us also went in.

It was not a large room, and the five of us—myself, the patient rep, the chaplain, the nurse, and the young man's mother—found ourselves standing in a circle around the young man's bed. His mother looked silently at his face. After a moment, the chaplain asked if she would like him to say a prayer. She nodded, and we all held hands in our circle and bowed our heads.

I don't remember the prayer. I know that it was not long, but long enough, and that it invoked no dogma other than a faith in, and assurance of, the love of God, as well as a hope for a peaceful passing into God's care.

When he had finished, the mother nodded and said thank you. Then, as the rest of us stood silently, she began to talk to her son. Once more she told him that she loved him. She told him that his baby boy was doing fine, and that his girlfriend missed him, often came to see him, and was taking good care of the child. She promised that she herself would continue to look after the two of them and help raise the child. Then she told him again that she loved him, always.

When the mother had been silent for a moment, the nurse stepped out of the circle, got the chair from the corner of the room, and put it next to her, inviting her to sit, which she did, still holding her son's hand. I waited a moment, then asked her if she needed anything more from me. She shook her head no and said thank you. I said I would be seeing other patients but I could come back immediately anytime, and then left the room.

It did not take long. About forty-five minutes later, the nurse came to tell me that his blood pressure was dropping and his breathing was becoming irregular. I went back to his room and found the patient rep sitting at the back-hall nurses' station. She looked up and said that the mother had wanted to be alone so she had stepped outside.

I opened the door a little way, just enough to see her without entering. She sat silent, looking at her son and holding his hand. The young man's breathing was indeed irregular, a pattern of rapid deep sighs, followed by long pauses of a half minute or more, gradually getting longer. The name for this is Cheyne-Stokes breathing, and it is a sign of imminent death.

I asked if she needed anything, and whether she understood what was happening. She nodded without speaking. I said that if she wanted any of us, we would be right outside. Then I closed the door as softly as I could.

In a few minutes it was over. It had been peaceful and—I think—without physical pain. Sir William Osler, a famous physician of the early twentieth century, referred to pneumonia as "the old man's friend" because it seemed an easy way to die. Perhaps it was for this young man as well.

Afterward we met with his mother again. Her questions were mostly about what she had to do next. When she finished, she thanked all of us and left. I don't remember what I did then, but I'm sure that I went up front, picked up the next chart in the rack, and went to see the patient.

That was my job.

CHAPTER TWO

Shears

I REMEMBER THAT it was summer. I know that, because I know I was a third-year medical student on my first clinical rotation, which happened to be surgery, and that it took place in the first three months of the school year, from July through September.

Also, I remember that it was hot.

Today an urban city hospital is a tall building made of steel and glass, with tiled hallways and automatic elevators that slide silently between the floors. Often the windows do not open, and the temperature is maintained at a constant level every day of the year, winter and summer.

But this was fifty years ago, and hospitals were different. The Boston City Hospital that lives in my memory was not glass and steel but concrete and brick. Heat was provided in the winter by radiators, which clanked and banged when the hot water was turned on. As for the summers, I don't recall whether the hospital had any air-conditioning other than those bulky boxlike contraptions that sat in the window and made propeller noises as they blew cold air into the room. It was a Saturday, late morning. It must have been after morning rounds, and I might have been taking a break from the little scut-work chores that medical students were assigned to do. I recall that I was sitting and drinking coffee when the junior surgical resident on our service put his head through the door and said, "Let's head to the OR. The emergency room has a guy who got stabbed in the back of his neck."

I'm sure I got up in a hurry; this was the sort of stuff medical students lived for. Once in the OR, I stood by the wall with the other third-year student so we wouldn't be in the way.

My memory of the OR is interesting, if only as a good example of how our memory actually works—or fails to. What I have is not one memory but two memories that coexist. The first is a vague sense that the room was a dull gray, with an OR table in the middle and steel shelves along the walls. That's what ORs looked like—and many still do.

But overlaid on that memory is another one, more powerful. In that other memory, the ceiling of the OR is a large glass skylight. The room is filled with sunlight. There are wooden workbenches on the sides of the room, holding gardening tools, and green plants with vines climbing up the walls toward the sunlight. I'm sure I have this utterly false memory for the simple reason that the man who had been stabbed was a gardener.

He was middle-aged, dressed in faded denim coveralls, solid work shoes, and a worn and dusty plaid flannel shirt.

He had been at work when it happened. Evidently a coworker had attacked him. I don't remember why or even whether I ever knew why. (I usually don't remember the reasons people are attacked for the simple reason that they never seem to make any sense.) But it must have been a spontaneous act of rage. After all, who in their right mind would premeditate stabbing someone in the neck with a pair of pruning shears?

As we waited, the ER nurse wheeled him into the room. He wasn't lying on a stretcher but sitting upright in a wheelchair. At first I didn't see the shears; the door to the room was facing us, and from the front there was nothing to see. But she pushed him forward past the foot of the OR table and then turned him right, stopping alongside it—and there they were. He sat motionless and rigid, staring straight ahead. It was as if he were some kind of grisly windup toy, with a key in the back of his neck shaped like the handle of a pair of shears.

Given how it had been done, the work of his assailant had been a marvel of precision. The shears were closed, the two handles touching each other, making the two blades functionally into one. Obviously, he had held it like a knife, his hand around both handles at once, as he drove the blades deep into his victim's neck. His aim could not have been more perfect: the shears were embedded in the midpoint of his neck, halfway from his shoulders to the back of his head. They were also exactly in the midline, not even a little to the right or left. Finally, they stood out from his neck at almost exactly ninety degrees, with the flat sides of the blades parallel to his spine.

Yet with such an injury, how could he look so well? The blades could not have been shorter than a few inches, and the shears were not taped in place. They had clearly penetrated deeply enough to sit stable and firm in the wound. But they were aimed directly at his spinal cord. How could he be sitting upright, breathing, holding on to the armrests of the chair? How could he still be alive?

No one wasted any time. Immediately the senior surgical resident bent down by the wheelchair and began to question him. The man had been sitting motionless, his fear written in his face, but asking no questions, either about how badly he was hurt or about whether he was going to die. Even so, when the resident began asking him the basic questions—How was he feeling? When had he last eaten? Did he have any significant medical problems?—he answered readily, with simple, short answers.

He asked no questions himself. It was as if he did not want to hear the answer to the important question; he would know it soon enough. We were all sweating a little just from the heat, and he was sweating too. I seem to remember him asking if someone would wipe his face, even though he knew he could move his hands. The nurse complied.

He could indeed move his hands—and his feet. That surprised me. His grips were strong, and when asked to do so, he could stand. The two surgical residents helped him of course, and then assisted him to sit on the table, which had been lowered to allow him to do so. Then they supported him as he turned and lay down, face forward. The front of the table had been lowered even further, and part of it removed so that it supported his face the way massage tables do. Thus, quickly and easily, he was resting facedown, with the shears sticking upward. He lay that way, patient, still without questions, waiting with us for the person who might save him to arrive.

The neurosurgeon had to come from home, but he did not

take long. When he came into the room, he had the X-rays that the ER staff had taken, and he slipped them deftly and expertly into the clips that bordered the screen. (It's harder to do than it looks, and it became apparent to us early that being graceful at snapping X-rays into place on a view box was another of the subtle ways for us to display our competence.)

When we looked at the films, everything became clear—and terrifying. On the one hand, it was one more example of the perfection of the blow. Not merely had it struck exactly in the midline, exactly halfway up the neck, and with the blades exactly parallel to the spinal column, but the point of the blade had exactly and precisely penetrated just between two of the bones in his neck and stopped just before entering his spinal canal. So he was completely neurologically intact, as if nothing had happened.

Intact? Well, yes, in the way a person strapped into a bomb is completely intact—until, of course, the bomb goes off. The problem was that bones are not just bones. They are filled with blood vessels, arteries, veins, even bone marrow. And when you cut into them, they bleed—a lot. At the moment, there was no evidence that this man was having any significant bleeding, certainly not into his spinal column. But was that simply because the blades themselves were putting pressure on those blood vessels? If so, then what? The shears could not be left in place, and if they were all that was preventing the bleeding, what would happen when they were removed?

The neurosurgeon looked at the films carefully for a minute or two. Then he shrugged his shoulders and said, "Well, I guess I have to take the damn thing out."

Then he turned and told the residents and the nurses to get ready for an emergency decompression and fixation of the cervical spine. This was surgery talk for opening the back of the patient's neck, then sucking out the blood as fast as he could, at the same time using cautery and tiny clamps to stop all subsequent bleeding—doing this while avoiding further damage to the spinal cord or the nerves coming out from it— and then tacking any broken bone fragments together with screws until everything was, maybe, good again; and doing all this *right now*. He could do that sort of thing.

And so they all got ready. The anesthesiologist was called and quickly set up to provide emergency anesthesia—though how he would do so with a patient who was lying facedown with a broken neck I could not imagine. At the same time, the neurosurgical operating tool kit, full of odd-looking clamps and things that might have been special saws and drills, as well as the usual scalpel handles and retractors, was brought and opened.

Equally important, while this was going on, one of the surgical residents sat by the patient's head and explained to him as best he could what was happening and what they might have to do. Once more—and I'm sure the resident was very relieved by this—the patient asked no questions, and after giving verbal agreement, he even reached up with his right hand to physically sign the form. As he did so, I found myself wondering if that was the last time he would ever move that hand.

When those preparations were complete, the nurses washed his neck—carefully so as not to disturb the shears. They had previously cut off his shirt, but they left his pants and shoes on simply to avoid unnecessary motion. Finally, he was draped so that the shears were sticking out of a hole in the cloth.

Only then was the neurosurgeon ready. He had placed a small footstool by the patient's head so that he would have as much leverage as possible as he pulled out the shears. He stood on it, then turned slightly and addressed the patient. "Sir, I'm going to take this thing out now. As I do, I need you to do something for me: if you start to feel anything unusual in your neck or your arms or hands or feet, any pain or tingling or anything, I want you to tell me right away. Can you do that?"

"Yes, sir," said the patient, still without moving.

None of us moved. I don't think any of us were even breathing. The neurosurgeon got a good grip on the shears. Then he took a deep breath and pulled.

At first nothing happened. He stopped, readjusted his grip, and pulled again, still firmly but also slowly and evenly, without any evident hurry. This time the scissors slid from the wound, and he placed them on the tray.

Then he said, "I have the shears out now. How are you feeling?"

For the first time, the patient moved without being told to do so. He lifted both his hands and wiggled his fingers. "Fine, sir," he said.

The neurosurgeon nodded. Then he asked, "Can you wiggle your feet?"

For a moment, nothing happened. Then, slowly, the drape that covered the patient's legs began to wiggle.

The neurosurgeon stood quietly for a moment, looking down at the now-empty hole in the patient's neck. He glanced almost casually for a moment at the moving drape and then turned back to the wound and examined it closely. Without looking up, he held out his hand. "Swab on a stick, please."

The nurse had prepared several long-handled clamps, each holding a cotton sponge soaked in Betadine. She put one in his outstretched hand. Holding the wound open with his other hand, he peered inside, then swabbed it gently with the Betadine sponge. Then when he was satisfied that there were no significant objects in the wound or any major bleeding, he took a large syringe filled with a saline solution and flushed the wound out several times. He looked at it closely once more. "Seems okay," he said. "Let's close."

He held out his hand again, took a suture, and began to sew up the small laceration that remained.

So what happened? How is it possible that a patient could survive such an injury? Simply because it had been so amazingly precise. Human beings are bilaterally symmetrical. That means that in general, if you have something on your left side, you have another one in the corresponding place on the right.

But it means another thing as well: there are very few structures that cross the midline. It is true that there are a great many blood vessels in the vertebrae—but they are all on one side or the other. The shears had gone precisely between them: the blood vessels, the ligaments and supporting structures, even almost all the bone—and then stopped before reaching the one structure that is truly midline: the cord itself.

It happened a half century ago. And I have never seen anything like it since.

Well, perhaps one other time. But that comes later.

CHAPTER THREE

The Intensive Care Nursery: Baptism

I DID NOT start out to be an emergency physician. For one thing, in those days there was no such thing. Teaching hospitals staffed their ERs with residents and medical students. Private hospitals were staffed in rotation by the members of the medical staff, regardless of specialty. I had enjoyed my time in the Boston City Hospital Emergency Room during medical school, but it never occurred to me that I would spend my life in such a place.

I wanted to be a pediatrician.

So on July 1, 1968, I began my pediatric internship at the University of California, San Francisco Medical Center. I spent my first month working on the general pediatric floor. There I assisted with the care of sick children, many of whom were afflicted with diseases I had never seen before and have not seen since; such is the nature of an academic referral hospital. Then, on August 1, feeling experienced and well prepared, I began my two-month rotation in the intensive care nursery, otherwise known as the ICN.

Please remember that, before arriving at the ICN, I had spent four years at a reasonably reputable college studying science, history, literature, and all the other things that universities thought were essential prerequisites to being an educated person, and which medical schools thought were essential prerequisites to being admitted. After that, I entered an equally reputable medical school. There, for the first two years, I studied all the science that they believed to be true at that time, and for the last two years, I followed real doctors around the wards, assisting them in their work. Finally, I had just finished a month on the general pediatric floor helping to take care of some very sick children. Therefore, you might think I would be well prepared to take care of little babies. I certainly thought so.

It would be hard to overstate how wrong I was.

Oh, I knew a lot of things: pharmacology, pathophysiology, anatomy, and all that other stuff that doctors have to know in order to do what doctors have to do. I had watched what doctors did, and even acted out the role of doctor under the close supervision of experienced residents, fellows, and attending physicians. (A resident is simply a physician in training who is a year or two ahead of the intern. A fellow is a physician who has finished residency but who is taking a year or two of specialty training before entering practice. An attending is the fully trained, credentialed, and experienced physician who, at a teaching hospital, is ultimately responsible for the care of the patients, and for supervising the fellows, residents, and interns who are helping him or her to carry out that responsibility.) But until the ICN, I had never quite experienced how it felt to *be* a doctor, to be on my own in critical situations, responsible for crucial decisions about a patient's care.

That doesn't mean I walked in a student and walked out two months later a doctor. It was the reverse. I started the ICN thinking I was a pretty smart doctor already, that I knew a lot and should be able to shine. I left knowing just how much of a student I still was and always would be; how little I—or anyone—knew about the human body; and how little we could do to reverse the damage that occurs when our bodies' natural processes go awry. It is not too much to say that everything I have seen and done over the nearly fifty years since—every success, every mistake, every regret—I tasted first in the UCSF intensive care nursery.

But why the ICN? Weren't these just a bunch of little babies? How could they have had time to get injured or sick? Why did these turn out to be the most desperately and uniquely ill patients I would ever see?

The reason is simple. The uterus, where babies spend the first nine months of their lives, is a place built entirely for their benefit. Unlike the outside world, the uterus has no other purpose than to keep a baby alive and thriving. A baby in the uterus need do nothing for itself to live and grow without any problem—not eat, not drink, not even breathe. Therefore, even if there are important organs in a baby's body that are malformed or do not work, the baby will do just fine. Until, of course, the moment it is born.

When that happens, the world changes completely—and immediately. Abruptly all those organs have to actually do what they are meant to do. Therefore, if any of them don't work perfectly, the child who depends on them can quickly become very sick. When this happens, it is one of life's greatest and least expected disasters. Confronting that reality is what neonatologists do for a living.

On that first day, I did not realize any of that. I knew it was going to be a hard couple of months. The hours alone were a killer—and indeed in later years such a schedule would not even be legal. There were two interns. Both worked every day, and we alternated nights. We did have a sleeping room, though I don't even remember where it was, much less what it looked like. There was also a third-year resident who supervised us. He—on all my ICN rotations, the resident and the other interns were male—was never off. He did go home each night, but he took his beeper with him, and if he ever slept a full night without at least one or two calls from us, I don't remember it.

Morning rounds were at eight o'clock, and when the attending arrived, we would already be there. The resident would be wearing a white jacket and pants, a white shirt and tie, and look showered and clean—regardless of how the night had been. The intern who was just coming on duty would be wearing white scrubs and a white gown, tied at the back, like the one patients wear, and would also look rested. He had doubtless slept long and hard the night before.

The intern who had been on duty all night would be dressed the same, but he would not look the same. He was usually unshaven, and his eyes were always red. Most obviously, the front of his gown would be covered with the marks of a ballpoint pen, where he had recorded the results of blood gas determinations, stat lab results, notes from phone calls, and other miscellanea. (We used our gown as scratch paper because it was a clean white surface that was always at hand, one that we knew we could not lose no matter how tired we were.)

We got used to working tired. If we got more than two or three hours of sleep on our nights on call, it was unusual. Mostly that seemed to work; sometimes it didn't. One early morning around three o'clock, I was writing a note on a premature baby with very severe lung disease, and I fell asleep sitting at the desk. As often happens to the sleep deprived, I immediately began to dream, and in my dream, the chief pediatric surgeon came in and told me that the baby needed a lung transplant right away. Suddenly we were in the operating room and I was watching as he did the surgery. But then my head nodded, and as I caught myself, I awoke. I quickly finished my note, got myself yet another cup of coffee, and continued with my work.

Later that afternoon, as I signed my patients out to the other intern before going home to sleep, we got to this baby's chart. As I summarized the issues, he rapidly scanned my note—and abruptly stopped. "What's this?" he asked, and handed it to me, pointing to the middle of the page.

There was the note I had written. In it, in a semilegible scribble, was a discussion of his blood gas reports and the respirator settings. Then there was a little trail of ink where my hand had unconsciously drifted, and then, rather neatly, the words "At that point, the patient was taken to the operating room."

That was all. I told him the story and then drew a single careful line through those words and wrote "error" beside them. Even so, I did point out to my associate that they were not really an error, as they were an actual report of what had been going on at the time . . . in my dream.

Rounds would start in the well-baby nursery. In those days, perfectly normal babies often stayed two or three days in the hospital, and we usually had a few deliveries each day. It varied of course. I remember sometimes having fifteen or twenty "well newborns" and occasionally having none.

Those rounds took little time. A word about each baby, a glance from the attending, sometimes checking respirations, skin color, alertness—that would be enough. The resident was expected to have gone behind us to be sure that, in our inexperience, we had not missed a heart murmur, a minor change in color, or some other subtle sign that this one was not as normal as we had supposed.

When we were finished there, the difficult rounds began. Whereas occasionally the well-baby nursery was empty, the sick-baby nursery never was. To be in the well-baby nursery, you had to have been born down the hall, but sick babies could be transferred in from anywhere in Northern California—and they could have anything wrong that you could imagine.

Most were simply premature. Infants are defined as premature if they are born before thirty-seven weeks' gestation or weigh below twenty-five hundred grams (about five and a half pounds). However, it was the babies who were under thirty-four weeks and fifteen hundred grams who accounted for most of the seriously ill infants. In those days, their mortality rate was forty-five times that of normal infants.

Still, most of them lived. Remember, in the United States, very few infants of normal gestation died, and forty-five times very few is still very few. At the same time, infants born before thirty weeks with weights under a thousand grams usually did not survive. And we always had one or two of those.

Nowadays sick newborns do much better—thanks in no small degree to the neonatologists who then were working at UCSF. While I was there, George Gregory, along with Rod Phibbs and Joe Kitterman, was inventing continuous positive airway pressure, or CPAP, a technique for keeping the lungs inflated and allowing for more oxygen exchange in the face of severely underdeveloped lungs. The impact this technique and its descendants has had, not only on neonatal care but on the whole field of respiratory and critical care, cannot be overstated.

We never knew what kind of day it would be. Occasionally we knew ahead of time that a problem baby was going to be born. But more than half of the sick newborns just got born, got sick, got worked up, and got admitted, and there was no telling when that would happen or how sick they would be.

My own personal record was on Christmas Eve 1968. I was not married then; I was substituting in the ICN so that the intern who was on his ICN rotation could be home with his family. That night there were three separate deliveries of babies under a thousand grams—at a time when we already had two babies with severe respiratory disease, one of whom went on to die that night. I remember, around four o'clock in the morning, going to each of the mothers' rooms, telling this one that her child had stabilized but that he was not yet out of the woods, the next that her child was doing well, the next that her child was quite sick and I would get her in to see him as soon as things were stable, and then the last mother that her baby had died. I didn't get to the sleeping room that night.

They weren't just preemies. Babies now and then are born with abnormalities of their heart and blood vessels that pose no problems in intrauterine life but are lethal after birth. Some babies have abnormalities of their digestive tract so that food cannot go through. Some have malformations of the kidney and urinary tract such that urine cannot form or cannot flow. The list goes on: there is no part of the body that, in a newborn infant, cannot be malformed. And therefore in the ICN, there was nothing out of bounds. While lungs and hearts were the main course, there was always an infant with something different, often something I had never heard of.

We had one such baby when I began my rotation. He was in fact the newborn son of the chief resident in surgery that year. He had been born a few days before I started. He was a normal-term baby in every way with a normal newborn exam—except that shortly after he was born, he began to turn blue. A quick measurement showed that his blood oxygen saturation—which should have been nearly 100 percent— was down in the eighties and dropping.

So he had an emergency workup.

His problem was something called transposition of the great vessels, and when I started my rotation, he had already had a "mustard procedure," which was at that time the state of the art in surgical revision. (It was an open-heart operation in the days when open-heart surgery was not routine for adults, much less for children.) It had left him with a good correction of his deficit but nonetheless still seriously ill, with a dangerous postoperative recovery period ahead of him. Even so, I remember that on my first morning rounds, we lingered on him as much because of his educational interest as for any feeling of imminent disaster. The rest of the morning was taken up with what I would learn was the usual routine of reevaluating infants and checking blood gases, respiratory settings, and other lab values.

And then it was lunchtime. The attending physicians were back in their offices and labs—nearby, but not in the unit itself—and the resident and the other intern were down in the cafeteria. I was left as the doctor covering the ICN.

Of course, there were also nurses in the unit, but I remember the nurse assigned to the resident's child as if in a photograph. She was tall, as tall as I was, with long brown hair tied up in a bun. She had long arms and hands and a face that I remember as expressive, vital, attractive, open, always smiling and laughing, full of things to say. I think she was my age or a bit older and had been a nurse in the unit for several years. We were talking about something or another when, with no warning, the child's heart slowed—and then stopped.

We looked at each other for a long second. Then she quickly unhooked his breathing tube from the respirator, replaced it with a manual ventilator bag, and began to ventilate him with one hand while beginning chest compressions with the other. (Does that sound like a lot to do? It is.) I was frozen in place. Everything I knew vanished from my brain. All there was in the world was the nurse and the dying baby.

She looked up at me silently for a moment. Then, in a calm and steady voice, as her hands continued moving gracefully, she said, "Dr. Seward, I think you want to order me to give him some epinephrine."

Suddenly my brain started working. "You are quite right, nurse," I replied. "Could you remind me how much epinephrine I want you to give?" Handing me the ventilator bag, she reached for the syringes that were standing in cups by the bedside and told me; and as I continued the bag ventilation and chest compressions, I repeated her words to her as she gave the medicine. Then I took a deep breath. "Now, can you remind me what I'm going to order next?"

The rest of the resuscitation was a smooth dance of hands, medications, and brief "reminders." The baby lived. And I learned something important about the practice of medicine.

Knowing the responsibilities that come with your role is an essential part of what we do; after all, the buck must stop somewhere. But there is another truth that is just as essential. Like everyone else, I have blind spots and bad days. Therefore, in a situation in which mistakes are catastrophes, if I am missing something, and it is my good fortune that someone else in the room knows something I don't know, or sees something that I don't see, then it is crucial that I have already created a relationship with them so that it is easy and safe for them to help me, even if that means challenging what

I am doing. If they are wrong, it is my job to know that, to thank them for taking the risk of making the suggestion, and then to do what I think is right. But if they are correct—then someone might live who might otherwise have died.

CHAPTER FOUR

The Burden of Choice

NOT EVERYTHING IN the ICN was an emergency. Now and then there were tragedies that could not be fixed and yet would not go away; they just endured. Each day we would make our rounds, and ask ourselves what we could do to make this better. And each day we would have no answer.

Nothing made this more clear than the day we were called to the obstetrical OR for a C-section. An emergency cesarean section often meant a sick baby, and we had to be ready to assist the baby after it was delivered. This time the problem was that the baby was in a breech position and could not be turned, with a slowing fetal heart rate.

Most babies are born headfirst. This means that by the time the blood flow from the mother's placenta is pinched off, the baby already has his head out and can breathe. However, if the baby is born feetfirst—or, more commonly, butt or "breech" first, then the possibility exists that the blood supply will be cut off while the head is still inside. If at that point there are any problems with delivering the head, the baby may suffocate. Therefore, if examination shows the baby to be in breech position, the obstetrician will use their hands to push on the baby from outside, feeling its position through the mother's abdominal wall, in order to turn the baby headfirst. If the baby cannot be turned, the obstetrician will usually elect to deliver the baby by cesarean section to avoid the risk of breech delivery.

This mother had not had much prenatal care, and her presentation to the emergency room was the first time she had been seen at UCSF. In addition, the obstetrician had tried several times to turn the baby but had been utterly unable to do so. Finally, the baby's heart rate had begun to drop—a serious sign that it was not getting enough oxygen. Therefore, quite correctly, the obstetrician had chosen to do a cesarean section. As he did so, the senior resident and I stood by.

The operation was simple and uneventful. The mother was put to sleep, a horizontal incision was made in her lower abdomen, and another one in her uterus. The amniotic fluid splashed out and was quickly sucked away, and the obstetrician reached in and removed the baby.

That was when it stopped being routine.

The obstetrician held the baby for a few seconds, staring at him. Then, without speaking, he turned and handed him to the resident, who also said nothing as he placed the baby into the bassinet, absentmindedly and as a habit, drying him with a towel. As he did so, he quietly said, "Holy shit." It sounded like a prayer.

Then he asked someone to page the attending neonatologist.

I stood by the bassinet and looked at the child lying there. From the neck down he certainly was a child, normal in every way. However, from the neck up—well, it was easy to see why he was a breech baby that could not be turned.

At the front of what had to be called the head was a small, misshapen face. However, above and behind this face, instead of a skull was something that looked like a large pink watermelon. Later, when the dust settled, and the X-rays and ultrasounds were done, they confirmed what our brief examination had already told us: that the development of this child's nervous system had gone terribly wrong, and that it had done so in two ways.

First, he had a condition called anencephaly, or in English, "no brain." In simple terms, his brain was not merely damaged; it had never formed at all. What he did have was that part of the nervous system that controls automatic functions—breathing, heart rate, basic motor reflexes, and so on. Therefore, he could breathe and have a heartbeat. In fact, because most of the activities of a newborn are reflexive, he could in many ways act like a normal newborn.

What he lacked was any hope for developing any ability to do anything more. Furthermore—to the best of our knowledge then and now—he lacked the ability to experience even the little that he could do. Children with this anomaly usually do not even survive the pregnancy. Those who do invariably die in the first few days of life.

The second condition he had is called hydrocephalus, or water on the brain. In most anencephaly, the back of the head does not close. The small amount of nervous tissue he does have is open and exposed to the world. However, in this case, the head had closed—perhaps offering some protection to the fragment of nervous system he possessed—and didn't allow for any release of spinal fluid. Therefore, the fluid had continued to collect, inflating the area where the brain might have been, turning the baby's head into a giant water balloon.

The child did not cry or move much. I confess that I found myself hoping that he would not breathe. In a normal delivery, at this point we would have been vigorously drying the baby, both to keep him warm and to stimulate him to cry. But neither of us made a move to do so.

We knew that this child could not live for more than a short time. We thought it had to be true that there was nothing in the child's brain that was conscious and therefore capable of experiencing pain or discomfort. But we could not be completely sure. Science cannot, even now, answer with complete certainty the question of what constitutes consciousness.

Nonetheless, even without a functioning brain, his primitive reflexes still existed. After what seemed like a very long time, we saw one short breath, then another, and another. Then the baby's color began to turn from pale white to blue to pink. The resident listened to the heart and lungs, which were normal, and then together we wheeled the bassinet to the newborn nursery.

The attending, Dr. Tooley, arrived immediately, and when the baby had been evaluated and the diagnosis made, he sat with the parents for a long time, explaining what had happened and what the issues were. Then he explained their options, one of which was to simply walk away. That was what they chose. We never saw or heard from them again. So it fell to Dr. Tooley to preside with dignity and care over the remaining days of the life of this profoundly damaged child.

Some readers will wonder whether this was legal. I was

not present for any conversations Dr. Tooley had with social services and child protective services, or with the judge and guardian ad litem. However, as the death of abandoned children was a sad but normal part of life in the ICN, I am certain that he followed whatever protocols the law required.

I do know that Dr. Tooley was legally empowered to decide what to do. Furthermore, in my opinion, there was no other mechanism that would have led to better care or better decisions than the ones Dr. Tooley made. Doctors are not gods. But sometimes they are required to clean up life's messes, because there is no one else who can.

Dr. Tooley was then the chief of neonatology, with a little over half a lifetime of dedicated service to sick newborn children and their families. He was tall and thin, and he walked, moved, and used the English language with gravity and elegance. If he had done patient rounds wearing a white tie and tails, he would not have appeared out of character. Shortly before I began my rotation, he had had a serious automobile accident in which he had broken the thigh bone of one of his legs—I don't remember which. Therefore, for my entire rotation, he conducted his rounds on crutches.

On anyone else, the crutches would have been a liability. For Dr. Tooley, they were an addition to his presence. He used them to walk, of course, but also as he lectured to us, he would lean on them like twin podiums, freeing his hands for demonstrations; he also used them to gesture, as a gentleman might use a straight cane.

The problem in this situation was that none of the things he could do so well were of any use. There was no test, no respirator setting, and no medication dose that could change a thing. And what was mercy? To try to lengthen this child's life? Or to allow it to be short? And how should we implement whichever we chose? Also, if by some chance this child could suffer, then was it suffering? How could we tell? And if it was, should we prolong it? Answering these questions was Dr. Tooley's responsibility, but it was not solely his. All of us, resident, interns, and nurses, shared the experience of caring for this child, even if Dr. Tooley held the final decision. So last of all, what was his responsibility to us, and ours to him?

His first decision was to put the baby in the well-child nursery, but in a part where he could not be observed by the parents and visitors of other children. Then during our morning rounds, we—that is, Dr. Tooley, the interns, the resident, and all the nurses involved in this child's care—would spend a few minutes looking at the child while we wondered what to do.

At first, when we expected him to die in a day or so, we treated him as we would a normal baby. Sucking is a primitive reflex, and while he did not suck well, he could do so sufficiently to take a little baby formula. So that is what Dr. Tooley asked the nurses to give to the child. But then a week went by, then ten days, and nothing changed. Yes, the baby lost some weight, but certainly most of that had to be from the massive reservoir of fluid in the sack of his head. Even so, he breathed, sucked somewhat, and lived.

One day "we" decided to stop feeding him. I say "we" because, while it remained Dr. Tooley's decision, we all participated in the discussion, and none of us disagreed. As we did not know whether the child could experience thirst, Dr. Tooley continued to order that he have water.

And we continued to wait. The time seemed endless, each day another reminder of our own powerlessness. I remember one morning when, as we were standing around the bassinet, someone said, "God, maybe one of us should just come in one night and give him a big dose of morphine."

We knew he did not mean it. We knew he had said such a thing only because he knew he was surrounded by people who understood that he was simply expressing the pain we all felt as we watched this tragedy take place. I think someone said, "I know what you mean," so he would know that he was not alone. But otherwise no one said anything.

The next day—I think it had been nearly three weeks— Dr. Tooley said, "How would you feel if we stopped giving this baby anything to drink?" None of us replied, so Dr. Tooley continued. "Instead, we will give small amounts of morphine to make sure he is not in any pain and is not thirsty." There was a murmur of agreement. And I know that I took a deep breath and nodded.

It did not last long. Three days later when I came in for rounds, the bassinet was empty. I looked at the nurses and asked them when it had happened. They told me that it had been the middle of the night. I asked them how they all were. They nodded that they were okay, and one said she was very glad it was over. Then we went on with our rounds.

Dr. Tooley died in 1992. The ICN is now named the William H. Tooley Intensive Care Nursery.

CHAPTER FIVE

Hands

I HAD THE privilege of watching Dr. Alfred A. de Lorimier operate a few times, and each time it amazed me that, even when operating on patients who were smaller than one of his large, thin-fingered hands, he could do the most incredibly delicate and precise work, all the while telling stories of sailing on San Francisco Bay. I remember once watching him operate on a premature baby, part of whose bowel had died from infection. The bowel wall was as thin as the rubber of the gloves he wore, with the diameter and consistency of a piece of overcooked macaroni—and yet with swift and effortless strokes, he cut away and removed the dead bowel, and then, with unimaginably tiny stitches, he sewed the two living ends together.

He even operated on me once. I had a small recurrent cyst over my left collarbone that occasionally would swell and drain, and I was concerned that it might prove to be a source of infection in the nursery. I asked him if he thought so, and he said, "Let me see." He pulled down my collar for a second and then said, "Got a minute?" I nodded, and almost before I knew what was happening, I was lying on my back in a procedure room as he excised the entire cyst, in one piece. It never recurred, and I have the scar as a souvenir.

But the most delicate operation I ever saw him perform, and the one that most clearly showed me what kind of a human being he was, happened early one afternoon in the ICN. It had been an ordinary day, if such a thing can ever be said of that place. There were several small recovering preemies in the nursery, all doing well and gradually gaining enough weight to go home.

There was one in particular who, even after a couple of weeks, in a unit that was designed for tiny premature infants, was still the smallest child there. As I recall, Dr. de Lorimier had already operated on her once for a gastroschisis (a failure of part of the front abdominal wall to develop, leaving the child with a hole through which some or all of her abdominal organs protrude into the outside world), from which she was recovering well. She no longer had umbilical lines, and her only intravenous line was in the back of her right hand—a thin plastic tube that had been magically inserted into a vein no larger than a heavy silk thread, in a hand that, from wrist to fingertip, would fit on a postage stamp. Then, to stabilize the IV line, the baby's hand was clenched around a small cotton sponge, wrapped in gauze, and taped to a wooden tongue depressor.

The nurse caring for her that day was, for my money, one of the best. She had been in the ICN for a couple of years and loved her job. She was cheery and bright and could spot a subtle change in the color or breathing of a sick preemie way before I could and get the help needed in time for it to do some good. Like my friend from the first day, she made working in the ICN seem both safe and enjoyable.

So I was shocked when I heard her scream, "My God! Her thumb! I cut off her thumb!" I couldn't believe that I had heard her correctly. How could she cut off a child's thumb? How could such a thing even be possible?

But she had. She had been doing something she did every day—changing the dressing that covered the IV and held it in place. To do so, she had inserted a pair of small bandage scissors under the dressing and away from the fingers, over on the side of the wrapped gauze, and cut through it so that it could be unwrapped. But today the child's thumb had not been next to the other fingers but pointing away, like a hitch-hiker or an umpire calling someone out, and her scissors had cut it off.

Now she held the cotton gauze out to me. For a second I didn't see it, but then there it was, a tiny glob of tissue perhaps two or three millimeters long at the most. It looked for all the world like a tiny tidbit of chicken that might be left on a chopping block after trimming.

I looked at her. I don't remember what I said—probably something stupid like "It's going to be okay." Then I called the attending. I don't remember who it was, but when he answered I said that we needed a hand surgeon. He asked me why, and I told him. "You don't need a hand surgeon," he replied. "Call Al de Lorimier."

For a moment, I was puzzled. It was a hand injury; don't you get a hand surgeon? I thought Dr. de Lorimier just did general pediatric surgery, which meant abdomens. "No," said the attending, "he doesn't do abdomens; he does children. And it's his patient." Chastened, I paged Dr. de Lorimier.

He was there in a matter of minutes. I don't remember his exact words. I do remember that he was calm and concerned; not smiling but not showing any anger. We had placed a dressing over the place where the thumb had been and left the thumb itself lying on a piece of moistened gauze on a metal stand next to the baby. Dr. de Lorimier went over to the child, lifted the gauze, looked at it, and then closely inspected the tiny scrap of meat that was the thumb.

Then he looked up at the nurse. Her eyes were red, but she stood firmly by the baby. "This was you?" he asked. "Yes," she said, nodding, waiting, like a prisoner before a judge, for him to say whatever he would say. What he said was simply, "Okay, I want you to assist me. Can you set up for a laceration repair?" She nodded without speaking and went to get out the kit.

I would like to say that I watched him reattach the thumb. But I can't say that I really saw anything at all; it was too small. What I saw were his hands with those long, steady fingers gently holding the bit of tissue with some tissue forceps while placing impossibly small sutures in a circle around the thumb, binding it to the baby's tiny hand. All the while he talked quietly to the nurse. I don't know if I even heard what he said to her. I have an impression that sometimes he would ask her for an instrument, or some suture material or a saline flush. And sometimes he just said words of reassurance—that she was a good nurse; that this kind of thing could happen to anyone. I do know this: not once did he utter a single word of condemnation.

I wish I knew how it turned out. I don't know if the thumb stayed attached or if it dried up and died. I don't even remember if the child lived to go home or not. And I don't remember what happened to the nurse. I have a vague feeling that she left the ICN shortly after, but I can't be sure.

I do know that I have never forgotten the moment the accident occurred, or the sight of that insignificant morsel of tan flesh that had been destined to become a thumb. I have never forgotten the nurse and the astonishment and horror on her face at what she had done. And I have never forgotten the skill and humanity of Dr. Alfred de Lorimier.

CHAPTER SIX

Snap Judgment

EARLIER I NOTED that I did not plan to be an emergency physician; I had set out to be a pediatrician. So in the summer of 1974, after I finished my residency, my wife, Linda, and I packed two dogs, one cat, and everything we owned into a couple of cars and a U-Haul and moved north from San Francisco to Ukiah, a small town in Mendocino County, inland on Route 101. There I started working for two pediatricians about ten years older than I, who were partners in an office just outside of town.

In those days, there was no such specialty as emergency medicine and therefore no such thing as an emergency physician. There were no emergency departments; there were only emergency rooms, or ERs. Similarly, there was no special training required of the physicians who worked in the ER. In fact, "covering the ER" was an onerous duty required of all physicians on the hospital medical staff in rotation, regardless of their medical specialty.

They didn't usually do much treatment. What they really did was come to the hospital, examine the patient, decide what kind of doctor the patient needed, and call that person in. The system worked—sort of—partly because in those days there wasn't enough known about the initial management of critical illness and injury to realize how important training and experience in such care could be.

But then things changed. By the mid- to late seventies, emergency rooms were getting busier, and quality and liability problems were increasing. More and more hospitals found that they needed physicians who were willing to devote more time to covering the ER. For that reason, several large businesses started up that offered to provide outside doctors to staff hospital emergency departments. They were mostly residents—doctors in training, as I had been at UC Medical Center.

But some of the physicians who had been covering the ER as a duty found that they liked it, and began working there not in addition to their regular medical practice but instead of having one.

I was one of them. I had been working in the ER part-time for three or four years when, one afternoon while working in our front yard with my wife, I suddenly said, "Why don't I just quit pediatrics and work in the ER full-time!" Something in my brain clicked, and pretty much on the spot, the decision was made. Emergency medicine and I were both in the same boat. No one had planned to create a new medical specialty, and I hadn't planned to practice it. But emergency medicine, which had hitherto been just a little tributary in the waters of medicine, was quite rapidly becoming a fast-flowing river of its own, and early on I fell in. And thereafter, when someone asked what I did for a living, I no longer answered that I was a pediatrician. I said that I was an "ER doc," for that was what we were called.

It was not a compliment. The profession of ER doc confused many orthodox physicians. After all, why would anyone want to work at all hours in such a place? There must be something a little off about such a person. Perhaps some character flaw. It was like running off to be a cowboy or joining the circus. Or maybe they were just paying too much alimony.

But over the next twenty years, the increasing numbers of physicians who chose to work full-time in the ER because they liked doing so began to develop a body of knowledge specific to that arena. Articles were written; textbooks were published; a national professional association—the American College of Emergency Physicians—was established; residency programs were started; and a specialty board examination that awarded board certification in emergency medicine was instituted. Some did excellent academic research, which revolutionized trauma care, resuscitation, and airway management, to name only a few.

As all that happened, we gradually stopped being ER docs and became emergency physicians, who practiced the specialty of emergency medicine. At the same time, our workplace stopped being the ER and became the emergency department.

It was not an easy process. The emergency physicians who led that process, most of whom are now retired or deceased, are justly remembered as heroes of our specialty.

Nowadays most emergency physicians don't like to be called ER docs either. Instead, they refer to their workplace as the emergency department, not the ER. This is appropriate; they have earned a higher honorific. We aren't cowboys anymore.

Therefore, this is the point at which I must apologize to my peers. Throughout this book, I have chosen to refer to the place where I have practiced medicine for much of my life as the ER. Why is that? First, for better or worse, thanks to television and the movies, when we talk about the place where people with emergencies are cared for, *ER* is the term that most people understand. Second, we have learned from our surgery colleagues that our specialty may be organized as a department, but it is practiced in a room. Finally, please don't tell anybody, but late at night, in the privacy of my own home, I kind of like being an ER doc. It's fun to be a cowboy.

However, this story happened when I was still in pediatric practice and only occasionally visited the ER. In those days, we had some reasons for kids to be sick that no longer exist in this country. High on the list was a tiny organism called *Haemophilus influenzae*. You may have heard of it as "H flu." Nowadays virtually all children in the United States are immunized against it in infancy. But in those days H flu immunization was a distant dream.

We saw a lot of H flu infections. (I talk about H flu in the past tense. But it hasn't gone away. It's just that most kids are vaccinated against it so we don't see it often.) They happened in one of three ways.

Most commonly we saw it as children's ear infections. No big deal: Kid has fever, so look in the ears. If there is pus behind the eardrum, treat with amoxicillin. On to the next patient. (Antibiotic resistance? Never heard of it—not then.)

The second way H flu attacked children was much less common but a much bigger deal. It was one of the most common causes of meningitis. Now, that was an emergency.

You have most likely heard of meningitis. It's a fancy word for an infection of the meninges, the coverings of the brain. That's how it starts. But left untreated, in a matter of hours to a day or so, it can spread into the brain itself. Death—or serious and permanent brain damage—follows soon after. (Meningococcal meningitis, the one you hear about soldiers and college kids getting, is caused by a different organism. It is still around despite immunization and is more lethal.)

H flu meningitis wasn't common, but it wasn't rare either. I got used to seeing three or four cases of it each year, and my associates did as well. If you diagnosed it promptly and gave the correct antibiotics, most children did well. But it kept us on our toes.

There was one other bad trick that H flu could play. That's the subject of this story.

It was a weekend: it must have been, because weekends were the only time I would see kids in the ER instead of at the office. I remember the phone call from the boy's mother. She was worried. Her son—about four years old—had a fever. It had come on suddenly that day. And what worried her most was that his neck seemed to hurt and he didn't want to move it.

High fever, sick kid, and a stiff neck? That's meningitis until I know it's not, and I have a race against time. The sooner I get him diagnosed and get some antibiotics on board, the more likely he will do well. I told her to take him to the ER immediately and I would meet her there.

I got to the ER before they did. I told the nurse on duty what I was expecting and to set up for an IV and a lumbar puncture. The IV was for the antibiotics; the lumbar puncture, or spinal tap, was what we did to make the diagnosis. The infection is around the brain, and we can't stick needles up there. However, the fluid around the brain circulates down into the spinal canal, and a meningeal infection will be detectable there as well. This is the reason that people with meningitis have a stiff neck. The brain is inflamed, but so is the spinal canal, so moving it hurts.

I think most people have some idea how a spinal tap is done: The patient curls up in a ball. This bends the spine so that the space between the vertebrae opens a little bit, making it an easier target. Then we prep the lower back with an antiseptic and insert a needle between two of the vertebrae in the lower back, and into the spinal canal itself. Then we allow some spinal fluid to flow out into a tube, where we collect it and examine it to see if there are pus cells or bacteria or other signs of infection.

That sounds dangerous, but it's quite safe. The spinal cord ends around two-thirds of the way down the back, and all that is in the canal below that point are long, thin strands of spinal nerves extending downward from the cord. They are referred to as the cauda equina, or "horse's tail," because that's exactly how they look. The point is that the chance of accidentally sticking a needle into a spinal nerve is about the same as that of impaling a hair in a horse's tail. I couldn't do either if I tried.

The nurse was excellent. I remember her well. She had the LP (lumbar puncture) tray out, opened and ready, and was setting up the IV when the mother brought the child in.

I took them immediately to the treatment room and checked him over. I don't remember what his actual temperature was, but it was high. I remember him as pale and breathing rapidly. I asked him whether he could look down at his toes (a test for neck flexibility), but he would not bend his neck at all. I did not ask him to do more, but quickly told the mother that I was worried, that I suspected meningitis, and that I needed to do a lumbar puncture immediately. She nodded. He was already sitting on the table, so with the help of the nurse, I laid him down on his back, rolled him onto his side, and began to bend him into a curled-up position so I could do the tap.

The moment I did so, he stopped breathing.

And suddenly I knew what was really going on. And after all these years, it still ranks as one of the worst moments of my medical life.

Along with ear infections and meningitis, there is one other important infection caused by H flu. It is called epiglottitis, a quickly progressing infection of the epiglottis. Anatomically, the epiglottis is a leaf-shaped flap of cartilage, attached to the front wall of the throat, just above the opening of the trachea. It is thus a sort of trapdoor, one that shuts to keep you from inhaling your food when you swallow but opens when you are not swallowing so that you can breathe.

However, when an H flu infection comes along, the thin, flexible epiglottis swells up until it no longer resembles a leaf as much as a fat red thumb. And the more it swells, the more it blocks the opening of the trachea, making it harder and harder for the child to breathe.

So how do such children look when they present? Usually they have a fever. And they tend to look sick, unhappy, and frightened. They want to sit up because that makes it easier to breathe. As it becomes more severe, they tend to tilt their head back and lean forward while supporting their upper body with their hands. This posture, called tripoding, allows for the maximum opening of their airway.

Sometimes they make a raspy sound with each breath because of the narrowing of the windpipe. They also have a very sore throat, so sore that they don't like to move their neck. Partly that's because moving it makes it hurt more, but more important, bending their neck forward presses on the epiglottis, increasing the obstruction and making it harder to breathe.

In fact, fiddling with the epiglottis in any way in a patient with epiglottitis can cause an increase in the swelling and lead to disaster. For this reason, when a doctor suspects epiglottitis, she doesn't ask the patient to say "Ah" or put a wooden stick in his mouth to look inside. She doesn't give the child any shots or even take a temperature. She doesn't do much of any further exam at all.

Instead, she turns down the lights in the room and lets the child sit unmolested in the mother's lap, and does whatever else she can to keep the child as quiet and reassured as possible—while at the same time calling the ear, nose, and throat (ENT) specialist and telling him to get his fanny over to the hospital as soon as he can, take the child to the operating room, and with a special instrument called a bronchoscope, slide a tube into the windpipe and keep it open. When that is done, the child will breathe easier—and so will everyone else.

But that was not what I had done. Rather I had lain him down, folded him into a ball, and bent his neck forward toward his chest—in precisely the position he never should have been placed.

And now he was not breathing.

The moment that happened, every detail of what you just read abruptly filled my mind in a single giant flash of under-standing—including the realization that I had probably just killed him.

Now what should I do?

I did the only thing I could do: I rolled him onto his back, opened his mouth, positioned his head to open his airway as much as possible, put a respirator mask on his mouth and nose, and began squeezing the bag, to breathe for him.

I knew it wouldn't work; his epiglottis was occluding his airway. You can't ventilate a patient adequately through an obstructed airway without removing the obstruction.

Except, it turns out that—at least sometimes—you can.

Think about it. He was a four-year-old child. I was a thirty-two-year-old man. I was a lot stronger than he was. Also, he only had his diaphragm and rib muscles to breathe with, while I had both my arms and hands. He might not have been able to suck the air into his lungs past his swollen epiglottis, but I could sure as hell push it in.

So I did. At the same time, I asked the nurse to page the ENT doctor on call and then give the antibiotics through the IV. Then for another half hour, I stood there with the nurse and breathed for the child with a bag and mask.

The boy was fine with it. Before I started bagging him, he had been getting tired and scared, with increasing trouble getting his breath. Suddenly he didn't have to work anymore. Now he was getting plenty of oxygen. All he had to do was relax and rest on the gurney while his mother held him and while I squeezed the bag.

Soon enough the ENT specialist arrived. He had called ahead, so the OR team was ready. Off they went with the child. He was out of the hospital, completely recovered, in a few days.

For my part, I had learned two things. First, I learned that even if a patient can't breathe, it is still quite possible that I can breathe for him, particularly if the patient is a child. In fact, over the next few years—before H flu went away, taking childhood epiglottitis with it—I saw four or five more children with this disease, two of which I wound up having to bag because of a delay in getting an ENT specialist. They all did fine.

The second thing I learned was something I already knew, but now it had been carved into me as if with a chain saw. What I had done was the most dangerous thing a doctor can do: I had made a diagnosis without an adequate examination—in fact, even before seeing the patient. Therefore, when he came in to see me, I had noted all the things that I thought he should have with meningitis—fever, stiff neck, looking sick—ascribed his rapid breathing to his fever and illness, and failed to notice the things I was not expecting: the signs of respiratory obstruction. And those were precisely the findings that should have taken me to the correct diagnosis.

I could have killed him. I damn near did. I make diagnoses all the time. But now when I do, I try to remember the words of Oliver Cromwell, in a letter written over 350 years ago to the General Assembly of the Church of Scotland: "I beseech you in the bowels of Christ, think it possible you may be mistaken."

CHAPTER SEVEN

A Drowning

I HATE DROWNERS.
Not the people who drown; God, no.

What I hate is the random ripping away of the lives of—mostly—children. What I hate is having to look into the bewildered faces of their families and tell them that their child, who only a few minutes before was playing happily, has been taken away forever. And most of all, what I hate is that there is almost always nothing I can do to change things, no way to bring them back.

Didn't I go into this business to save lives?

It was early afternoon on a beautiful summer day. Of course it was; that's when children go swimming. And this was Ukiah, in Northern California, in the early eighties. In those days, it would have been hard to find a summer's day that was not beautiful.

I'm pretty sure it was a Saturday. The ER had been quiet that morning. That was no surprise; even people who don't feel well put off going to the ER on a beautiful Saturday morning. Also, the bike trips, the 10K races, the pickup football and rugby games had only just started, so the afternoon injuries hadn't happened yet. On such a day, if someone came to the ER, it was usually for something serious.

It was serious. The paramedic made that clear.

"Med control, this is Mendocino Ambulance. Please come in."

The radio was just a few steps away from where Jerry Chaney, the ER nursing director, and I were taking a break.

"This is med control," I replied. "Come in, Mendocino."

"We're about ten minutes out with a three-year-old girl. She was found down in the family swimming pool a few minutes ago. She is intubated and CPR is in progress. At the moment, she is unresponsive. Do you copy?" The words were painstakingly controlled and precise.

"I copy, Ukiah. Do you have a pulse or a rhythm? And do you know where the parents are?"

"Negative on pulse. Hard to interpret rhythm with CPR ongoing. The father is with us in the ambulance."

"Copy that. See you in ten. Med control out."

I hung up the radio. For a moment, Jerry and I looked at each other, saying nothing. Then Jerry took a deep breath and said, "I'll put her in bed one," and got up to get it ready. I went out front to ask the ward clerk to page the respiratory therapist and the X-ray tech.

In those days, Ukiah Valley Medical Center, where I was working, was a small hospital with a small ER. As such, the principal treatment area only had four stations, separated from one another by thin curtains. Bed one was the station closest to the entrance. The code cart, where we kept the equipment and medication required for most resuscitations, stood at the head of the gurney against the wall. Jerry tore off the small plastic ring around the latch that sealed the cart, removed the intubation and ventilation equipment, and set it near the head. Then he set up and hung two IVs.

I had returned by then, so I picked up a small hard board that had been leaning against the wall and laid it on the gurney. It was shaped vaguely like a child and was meant to make it easier for someone to effectively compress a child's chest during resuscitation. We covered it with a clean white sheet. Then we went together out to the ambulance entrance, where, in the heat and brightness of the day, we listened for the sound of the siren.

It wasn't ten minutes; it was only six or seven before we heard them. The sound came down Route 101 from Redwood Valley, then slowed as the ambulance turned off the highway and headed down Perkins Street into town. Barely a minute later, we could see it hurrying down Hospital Drive, and then onto the U-shaped driveway that in those days was the ambulance entrance to the ER.

The van had barely stopped when the driver jumped from the cab, ran to the back of the vehicle, and opened the rear door. Inside, the paramedic was doing single-person CPR. He continued chest compressions while we slid the stretcher out the back, lowered the wheels to ground, locked them in place, and rolled the child into the coolness of the ER.

The girl was dressed only in a damp bathing suit, which Jerry quickly removed, covering her with a warm blanket. At the same time, he lubricated an electronic temperature probe and slipped the end gently into the child's rectum. As he did so, I verified that the endotracheal tube, which the paramedic had placed into her windpipe so that we could breathe for her, was still in the right place, that it had not come out during the transport. I did it in the only way we could in those days: by listening carefully for good breath sounds on both sides, feeling the abdomen to be sure the stomach was not inflating, and watching for the rise and fall of the chest wall.

At that point, the paramedic stopped chest compressions for a few seconds while I felt for a carotid, brachial, or femoral pulse. (Neck, arm, and groin.) I did not find one. Then I checked her pupils with my flashlight. They were equal and dilated on both sides and did not respond to light. Lastly, I quickly examined the rest of her body for signs of physical injury and found none. The whole exam from start to finish took under thirty seconds. And during that time, neither Jerry, nor I, nor the paramedic or EMT, had noted any response of any kind to what should have been very uncomfortable procedures.

As we worked, I noted that the father had stayed with his child, refusing the invitation of the ward clerk to go out front to register the patient. He sat at the foot of the gurney in a chair that the ward clerk had brought for him and held the girl's feet in both his hands, rubbing them as if to warm them.

By then Jerry had the monitor leads in place, so I looked at the screen. There was some artifact from compressing her chest, but no clear sign of any electrical activity in the heart. I asked the EMT to pause chest compressions, and the line became straight. "Asystole," I said. It is the medical term for no heartbeat. "What's her temperature?"

That was a shot in the dark. People who drown in cold water can have a long period of slow and impalpable pulse and still occasionally recover, and it is sometimes worthwhile in such cases to prolong the resuscitation. The phrase used in the ER was "You aren't dead until you're warm and dead." But Jerry replied: "Thirty-six point five." In the more familiar Fahrenheit scale, it would be 97.7, or just a tiny bit below normal. I looked back at the screen, then at the girl. She was just a little younger than my son.

"Well, maybe it's fine V-fib. Let's give it a try. Start at fifty joules." Jerry nodded, and as I picked up the pediatric defibrillator paddles, he began to charge the machine. "Charging to fifty joules," he said.

I sometimes did that in those days when trying to resuscitate children. In asystole, the heart has simply stopped beating. That is obviously a bad thing in an adult, but in a child, it is even worse. Children have healthy hearts that will beat for a very long time even without any oxygen. That's the good news. The bad news is that when a child's heart does stop beating, it is because the lack of oxygen has been prolonged enough to shut down an otherwise healthy heart. Furthermore, because the brain is much more sensitive to the lack of oxygen than is the heart, asystole almost always implies that a lot of brain damage has already taken place.

Ventricular fibrillation, however, is something that a heart that is deprived of oxygen will do even before it is permanently damaged. The heart is still trying to contract; it's just that all the little bundles of heart muscle fibers are no longer doing so at the same time. Instead they are beating randomly and at different times. Therefore, the heart does not contract; it just wriggles.

On a cardiac monitor, this shows up as an irregular jagged line. A jolt of electricity fired through the heart during ventricular fibrillation can sometimes synchronize the muscle fibers again so their contractions will be effective. On the other hand, if ventricular fibrillation continues without being converted, the unsynchronized contractions will become weaker, and the jagged line becomes smaller and smaller until—sometimes—it looks a lot like the straight line of asystole—that is, no contractions at all. That is "fine ventricular fibrillation."

Fine V-fib is not a common rhythm. If it exists at all, it is one that occurs only when the heart is nearly dead. In children, it is particularly uncommon. In this case, when I called the rhythm on the monitor "possible fine ventricular fibrillation," it was not a considered medical judgment; it was an excuse.

We all knew the little girl was dead. At least Jerry, myself, the paramedic, and the EMT did. We had all seen drowned children too many times before not to know. I think the father knew also and was not letting himself believe it.

But we had only had her in our care for a minute or two, and this was a little girl, like our own children. We could not accept what we knew. And pretending that the heart might be in fine V-fib gave us an excuse to keep on trying.

So we did.

First we shocked her; we shocked her three times. Then we gave her IV epinephrine (adrenaline). That was the protocol for resuscitation in those days. We even had a little jingle to help us remember it: "Shock, shock, shock. Everybody shock. Big shock, little shock, little shock, big shock." The meaning of the jingle was to defibrillate up to three times (shock, shock, shock). If no organized rhythm returned, then give epinephrine and shock again (everybody shock). If there was still no return, then start medications that suppressed irregular rhythms—bretylium (big) and then lidocaine (little)—shocking again after each one. If that didn't work, reverse the order and repeat (big shock, little shock, little shock, big shock).

So we went through our little jingle and nothing worked. By this time about fifteen minutes had passed and we were out of protocol.

Actually, we were not quite out of protocol. There was a euphemistic phrase in the guidelines that went something like, "If no response, evaluate the advisability of discontinuing resuscitation." But nowhere in the protocol did it say directly what was so often the truth: "Pull yourself together. If nothing has worked by now, the patient is dead."

It was time to quit. I looked at Jerry, the paramedic, and the EMT. They looked back at me. Nothing needed to be said. I was the doctor. It was my call. So I turned to the father. I had only said a few words to him during the resuscitation, explaining what we were doing and what we hoped the medications might do. I'm sure I must have also said a few words about how sick she was, and how her failure to respond was a very bad sign. But now we were beyond bad signs.

"Sir," I said, "I'm so sorry to have to say this, but—"

He stopped me immediately. He was still at the end of the gurney, holding his child's feet. "No!" he said. "You can't quit. I know she's still here. I feel her. I know she's here in the room wanting to come back." As he said it, he looked up at the corner of the ceiling as if his daughter's spirit were floating there. He was crying now, still holding the child's feet, no longer paying attention to anything but his daughter—the daughter who had drowned while he had been watching over her.

Jerry and I looked at each other. I said, "Continue CPR." Then I got a chair and sat down next to the father, who stared at me and continued to cling to his child's foot. I asked him to tell me what had happened.

"I . . . I don't know," he said. He was now rubbing the girl's foot with both hands, as if the warming and chafing might awaken her.

"I mean, how did she come to be in the water?"

He looked up at me then, seeming slightly confused, as if his daughter being in the water were something he did not fully understand. As he answered me, his reply came in little chunks of words, almost as if they were stuck in his throat and he needed to cough them out as much as speak them.

"It was our pool . . . We have a Doughboy pool in the back-yard . . . She was swimming. I was watching her . . . I don't know how it happened . . . One minute she was fine and then . . . she was lying on the bottom of the pool . . . I jumped in and pulled her out." As he spoke, he stared at his daughter. He had stopped rubbing the pale, limp foot and was now gripping it hard, as if to drag her from the water again.

"What happened then?"

He looked up at me for a moment. "Then? Then I started pushing on her chest . . . Water came out of her mouth when I did it . . . I ran into the house and called 911. I told them what had happened and then I ran back out again. I kept on pushing on her chest till the ambulance came. She's going to be all right, isn't she?" The last sentence burst from him as if by accident, as if he had not meant to say it.

I thought, if he can't even let go of his daughter's foot, how can I ask him to let go of her life? How, for the second time that day, could I tear his child away from him as he sat there all alone?

I didn't answer. Instead I asked, "Where is her mother?"

He blinked a couple of times and thought for a moment. Then he said, "She's shopping . . . she went shopping . . . to the grocery store. To Safeway."

The ward clerk was still standing by. "Could you ask the police to see if they can find her?" I asked. She nodded and went back to her station to place the call.

I turned back to the man and said, "I'm sure we will find her soon." He nodded slightly. Then he said, "We moved here so she would be safe."

"What do you mean?" I asked.

"We were living in Los Angeles." He spoke softly, never looking at me, looking only at the pale child. "We thought the streets were dangerous. We came up here so she could live in a safe place." Then he was silent. I did not say anything. After a little while he said, "We only moved here a year ago."

I nodded. Then I looked at Jerry. He had just rotated off chest compression duty. I stood up and motioned to him to join me. We went over and stood by the door.

"I need a little advice," I asked.

"Okay," he said. Jerry had been an ER nurse for four or five years and the nursing director for over a year. He was also a religious man, one who carried his faith within himself and spoke little about it unless he was asked some direct question. He was a man who was comforted by his religion and able to give comfort and support to others. Now he was supporting me.

"This guy just had his daughter drown when he was supposed to be watching her," I said. "There is no way he is going to be able to tell us to stop. So we have a choice."

Jerry nodded.

"We can stop, despite anything he says, or . . ."

Jerry nodded again. He knew what I was going to say.

"Or we can just go on doing ventilation and compressions till his wife gets here and talk to her."

"That's fine with me," said Jerry. "But we are starting to have some other patients. Can we move her?"

"Of course," I said. "Let's move the whole operation to bed four and keep the curtains closed. No reason why anyone needs to be aware of it."

We both knew that from a strict medical point of view, it was futile. What I was asking him to do was to use staff time and resources in what was almost certainly an equally futile attempt to help a father with his grief. I don't know even now whether Jerry thought it was a good idea or not—or whether, as I said, he was just taking care of me.

I went back to the gurney and told the father that we would be continuing our resuscitation and would reevaluate the situation when his wife arrived. He nodded without saying anything. By then the paramedic and EMT had to go, so we borrowed a nurse from one of the inpatient services, along with the respiratory therapist, and explained what was happening. Then they went to relieve the ambulance people. As they did so, we moved the gurney over to the far wall and pulled the curtain. Now nothing out of the ordinary could be seen, and I could start to see the few patients who had checked in.

I don't remember how many there were; I don't remember what problems they had. In fact, I don't remember anything about them. But I do remember the arrival of the girl's mother about thirty minutes later.

She first came to the front desk, asking to see her child. I met her outside and told her that I would take her to her immediately but I needed to talk to her briefly before I did so. We went back to my office, but I don't think we sat down. I talked to her about the condition of her daughter. It was clear as I did so that she had already gotten it; the police had told her what had happened and she knew her daughter was dead. But how she felt about that was not my business. She would face that later in privacy.

Then I told her what we were doing, and I asked her what she wanted us to do next. She did not answer my question;

she simply nodded and asked to see her husband and her little girl. So I took her back to them in the ER.

She went to her child immediately and gently put her hand on her forehead. She stood there for a moment, silent and firm. I don't remember any tears. Then she turned to her husband. "They've done all they can," she said. "She's not here anymore. It's time to stop." He looked at her, tears in his eyes. Then he nodded and stood up. He may have said something, but if so I don't remember what it was. And then for the first time, he let go of his daughter. His wife hugged him, and then gently led him from the ER. I never saw them again.

CHAPTER EIGHT

The Heart Is a Pump

I T'S A SIMPLE idea for something so miraculous.

When I began my medical school course in cardiovascular physiology, "the heart is a pump" were the first words the professor wrote on the blackboard, and I have heard them—and spoken them—hundreds of times since.

The heart *is* a pump. But it is not an ordinary pump. First of all, it is a pump that is made up entirely of muscle. Moreover, that muscle is unique. It is not like the skeletal muscle found in your arms and legs and other moving body parts. Nor is it like the smooth muscle found in your intestines, around your blood vessels. Instead, cardiac muscle is made of a special kind of muscle cell that is found nowhere else in the body.

Cardiac muscle cells do look a lot like skeletal muscle cells. The principal difference is that skeletal muscle cells line up together to form a long series of parallel fibers that all pull in essentially the same direction. They are designed to pull on bones and bring them closer together.

Cardiac muscle fibers are, for the most part, not attached to anything but each other. Instead of parallel lines, they form a branching web of thousands upon thousands of crisscrossed muscle fibers linked together to form what is essentially a hollow ball of muscle, inside of which are four separate chambers. That muscle, like the piston in a gasoline engine, is not designed to pull on those chambers but to squeeze them and make them smaller.

But how does simply squeezing on those chambers pump the blood around?

First, the squeezing of the heart muscle is not like the hand of a boxer, squeezing all his fingers at once to make a fist. It is instead like the hand of a farmer milking a cow, who squeezes the teat first with his index finger, then his middle and finally his ring and small fingers, to push the milk down and out and into the bucket.

Similarly, in the heart, the squeezing starts first in the two upper chambers—the atria—which thereby push blood into the two lower chambers—the ventricles. Then, when the atria have finished squeezing, it is the ventricles' turn, pushing the blood out of the heart and on its way. Finally, just to be sure the blood goes in the correct direction, each chamber has a valve at the exit that opens when the blood pushes outward and closes when it tries to push back.

But why four chambers; why not just two? Because the blood doesn't pump the heart in a circle—out to the body, back to the heart. It pumps it in a figure eight, with the heart in the center, exactly where the circles touch. Remember the little baby in chapter three? It's as if we have two hearts pumping in two circles. One circle is to the lungs and back; the other circle is out to the body and back. But both circles originate from a single amazing ball of muscle.

Why amazing? It is not simply that its construction and mechanism permit this single small pump to push our entire blood supply through our lungs, then through our body and back again. It is also that, beginning well before we are born, it does that exercise approximately once every second for our entire life. That means that if we live roughly seventy years, our heart will have squeezed once a second, without a single moment of rest, considerably more than two billion times. If it were to stop for more than a second or two, we would quickly lose consciousness. If it did not start again within five or six minutes, our brains would die. We all know this. Yet like most everyday miracles, we take it for granted.

Until it doesn't happen.

My recollection is that he was fifty-three years old.

I don't know why I should remember something so specific; perhaps it's because he seemed too young to have such a terrible heart problem. After it was all over, I learned that until a few months prior, he had been perfectly normal and healthy. Then with no warning, he had suddenly suffered a severe heart attack, which, though he survived it, had left him with major damage to his left ventricle.

I also think I recall that he had required open-heart surgery on his coronary arteries—at the time a new and radical procedure. But that might be a false memory. After all, during our time together, I had more than ample time to look at his chest, and I don't recall seeing the long scar that is the badge of such surgery.

It doesn't matter. What does matter is that the damage to

his heart left him with permanent and severe heart failure. It also left him with the knowledge that he was a prime candidate for further problems. It was as if one day a bomb had gone off in his chest, nearly killing him, and then had left another bomb ticking inside him, waiting to explode.

I didn't know all that when he came in. When I first learned of his existence, all I knew was that the paramedics were bringing in a middle-aged male in cardiac arrest due to ventricular fibrillation.

At this point I'm sure I don't need to review what we did on his arrival. Either I or the paramedics intubated him, IVs were placed, drugs were given, and the customary electrical shocks were applied, to defibrillate him.

Then suddenly, surprisingly, it worked. On the monitor, in place of the random jagged lines of ventricular fibrillation, we saw the orderly peaks of a normal heartbeat marching across the screen.

But that was all. The patient remained unresponsive and we could not palpate a pulse.

There is a name for this. It's called pulseless electrical activity, or PEA. It's not that uncommon a situation for a badly damaged heart. It means that even though the heart is capable of normal electrical activity, and therefore produces a relatively normal heart tracing, the muscle fibers in the heart are so damaged that they cannot contract strongly enough to pump the blood around. In short, the monitor looks fine, but the patient has no functional heartbeat.

What one does in that case is simple: resume cardiac compressions, then try to figure out if the reason for this problem is something that we can fix. Perhaps he isn't getting enough oxygen; perhaps there is too much acid in the blood; perhaps there is fluid around the heart; or any of a number of things. So we started going through the list of possibilities. At that moment, I happened to be the person whose turn it was to do the compressions (they are hard work), so I started doing them again. That was when something totally unexpected happened.

He woke up.

His eyes abruptly opened, he began to move his arms, first up to his chest where I was pushing, and then toward his face.

I stopped chest compressions at once and grabbed his hands so that he could not pull out his endotracheal tube. Then I started to explain to him that he was in the hospital, that he had had a heart attack, that we had needed to put a tube into his windpipe to help him to breathe and . . . I realized he was no longer listening. Within a few seconds of my stopping chest compressions, he once more lost consciousness.

So I started them again. And once again he woke up.

It was obvious that he was awake. His eyes opened. He looked at me. His lips moved as he tried to speak, but he could not because of the ET tube. Once more, this time while continuing to compress his chest, I began to explain to him what had happened.

He understood me. I know that because over the next hour he nodded and shook his head appropriately (the ET tube still attached, as he was clearly on the brink of another full arrest, and I did not want to take the chance of not being able to breathe for him should that happen) as we talked about what was happening to him, what the possibilities were, and, ultimately, what we were going to do. I don't remember if he signed the consent forms, but his nods and shakes were very clear.

He understood what was happening to him. The question was, did we?

Almost immediately it was clear what the situation was. The tracing on the monitor was normal; his heart was electrically normal. And—probably—it was contracting a little bit. Our best guess was that heart valves were opening and closing correctly, making sure that blood flowed in the right direction. And his lungs were working. All that the heart needed to do its job was a little more force. And that was what our chest compressions seemed to be supplying.

Even so, he was clearly living on a knife edge. Whenever we stopped—which happened once or twice more before we fully realized what was going on—he lost consciousness, became unresponsive, and stopped trying to breathe. If we had stopped for more than a minute or two, he would have died. But otherwise he was awake, reasonably alert, and not in too much pain. We gave him some morphine, for which he expressed gratitude. After all, not only was his heart muscle hurting from the heart attack, but we were pushing on his chest about once a second. His brain, his lungs, and the rest of his body were working fine. His only problem was that his heart didn't work. And there was nothing we could do to fix that.

But there was one thing we could do. We could call for help.

I don't remember making the calls, or who I talked to. I know that it was the larger of the two hospitals in Santa

Rosa, a small city south of Ukiah, which had the closest major hospital. I must have spoken to the cardiologist on duty. I am sure that he was as surprised as I was at what was going on. But I remember being told that they would take him and see what they could do to help. They thought that perhaps an intra-aortic balloon pump might work. This is essentially a balloon at the end of a catheter that can be slipped into the aorta (the main artery coming out of the heart) via an artery in the groin. It can be made to inflate or deflate in time with the heart in such a way as to help the heart pump the blood.

But now we had another problem: how to get him to Santa Rosa? We knew that, however we did it, it had to be set up so that somebody could continue to do chest compressions nonstop all the way.

Our first idea was a helicopter. I'm not sure why that didn't work out. Perhaps it was unavailable, or perhaps the working space was not big enough. Both could have been true.

That left only one other choice: the ambulance in which he had arrived. The paramedics were available; it was full of gas. All that was needed was someone to push on his chest all the way down.

That was going to be me. After all, he was my patient. He was my responsibility. I was legally the highest-level medical person present. I needed to go.

And I wanted to go. How could I not?

I have thought of that trip often since then. The distance was sixty miles or so down a winding road, and I think they did it in a little over forty-five minutes. During that time, I must have taken turns doing compressions with one of the paramedics, but I can't be sure.

After all, my memory of that ride is not like a movie; it is like a photograph. I am kneeling beside the stretcher, my arms straight, and my hands on his breastbone, rhythmically compressing his chest. But I am not looking at my hands; I am looking at his face. He has reddish-blond hair. His eyes are open. They are blue. He is looking at me. I am talking to him, reassuring him, letting him know that I will not stop, that we will get him to Santa Rosa safely and that there would be experts to care for him, things that they could do. He is nodding, still looking at my face.

When we got there, he was still alive. They did take him to the ICU. There they did put in an intra-aortic balloon pump. And it worked: they were able to stop pushing on his chest, and they could take out the ET tube so he could talk.

He lived two more days. Later I learned that during that time, his family could see him, talk to him, and perhaps hold him. And they could say goodbye.

CHAPTER NINE

Colors

NOT EVERYTHING THAT happens in the ER is a story. Our encounters are usually too brief and limited. What they offer are snapshots with no stories—just images of people who are suddenly pulled out of their usual lives into a situation they could not previously imagine.

Here is one: a young man, sitting on a gurney, seeing beautiful colors.

I had been practicing for over fifteen years before I defibrillated a heart attack patient who was younger than I was.

That's not surprising. I graduated from medical school on my twenty-fifth birthday and finished my residency training five years later. I was in my early thirties when I began working in the ER part-time. By the time I turned forty, I had certainly treated my share of seriously ill patients, but the ones who were younger than me were generally ill from trauma, or from childhood cancer or serious infections—not clots in the coronary arteries.

It isn't that young people don't have heart disease. Autopsies performed back in the middle of the last century on American soldiers who were killed in Korea showed early fat deposits in the arteries of nineteen- and twenty-year-old boys. And I remember when I was in fifth grade, the father of a friend of mine dropped dead of a heart attack at thirty-five. That seemed old to me then.

I was due to see a young person try to die of a heart attack in front of me. I knew that. I also knew that heart disease is often missed in the young. So I tried to keep my suspicions up.

And one day he walked in the door.

He was in his midthirties; I think maybe thirty-six. He was not overweight; he did not have diabetes; he did not, as far as I could determine, abuse cocaine; and he exercised regularly. I don't think he even smoked.

Even so, the moment I began talking to him, he made me nervous. He told me that he had been feeling reasonably well, but for the last few days, he had been having some stomach discomfort. Okay, lots of people his age do.

But his stomach trouble was a little unusual. When he had it, he also felt a little short of breath. And one time he had broken a sweat.

There is a saying in the ER, "When the patient sweats, the doctor sweats." Sweating unrelated to exercise, being hot, or infection is a sign of the release of adrenaline in the body, which in turn is a response to some internal stress. I regard it with the same concern that I do an abnormal vital sign. The patient isn't going home until I know why he is sweating and that it isn't something bad, and sometimes not even then.

It did not take long to figure it out. That information alone was enough to prompt the nurses to take him straight to one of the cardiac rooms. When I got there, he was on a monitor, an IV was in place, a defibrillator was next to the bed, he had been given a couple of chewable baby aspirins and a squirt of nitroglycerin under his tongue, and he was getting extra oxygen by means of little tubes in his nose. The nurse had waited for me to arrive and then gone to get the EKG machine. So for a minute or two, I was alone in the room with him. I had just introduced myself and was asking those questions about his pain when he did something that proved beyond doubt that our worries were well founded.

He died.

No, he didn't really die. He did what, not many years ago, was considered to be the same thing: he went into ventricular fibrillation and his heart stopped pumping blood. I couldn't see his heart, of course. What I saw was that while talking to me, he suddenly gasped, his head fell backward onto the pillow, his eyes looked upward, and he became unresponsive. If that were not sufficiently convincing, his cardiac monitor suddenly showed only the chaotic wiggly line that was diagnostic of ventricular fibrillation.

I don't remember even thinking about what to do. As a reflex, I turned to the defibrillator, flipped it on, and started looking for the pads—these are large cotton squares soaked in a saline solution that are designed to protect the chest wall from being burned by the shock and still conduct the full charge across the heart.

I couldn't find them.

Later, of course, the nurse pointed them out to me, in plain sight in a pocket on the side of the defibrillator cart. That was no help; my wife will vouch for the fact that I have always been able to lose objects in plain sight. But a few seconds later, the defibrillator was fully charged, he was still in V-fib, and I still had not found the pads.

Oh well; no time to send out a search party. I grabbed the paddles, pressed the metal plates to his bare chest, and pushed the button.

It worked. Just like on TV. His body jerked, his arms flailed out, he gave a loud grunt, his eyes opened, and in the next few seconds he woke up. And indeed, now the monitor showed him to be once more in a normal rhythm. It was a quick recovery, but then he had been without blood to his brain only briefly.

By that time, the nurse was back with a couple of others to help, and we started pulling up syringes full of the medicines that block heart rhythm disturbances, so that he might not do it again.

But then he spoke.

"What was that?!" he said, in a voice filled with astonishment and alarm.

I put on my best doctor manner and replied that I was sorry if it had hurt, but his heart had just stopped and I had needed to give him a shock of electricity to start it again.

"My heart stopped?" He shook his head in confusion. "But that can't be."

"Why not?" I asked.

"I think I must have fallen asleep." He stopped for a second and briefly seemed annoyed. Then he said, "I was having such a wonderful dream."

Now this was the mideighties, around the time that reports of near-death experiences were just starting to be widely written about and discussed. For a moment, all the nurses in the room stopped what they were doing and looked at him. So did I.

I had to ask. "What were you dreaming about?"

He shook his head in confusion. "I don't remember exactly. All I know was that I was in such a wonderful place. And it was filled with such beautiful colors."

No one said a word.

Then he looked down at his chest where two large red paddle-shaped marks were starting to form. For a moment he looked upset. "And then . . ." he said, "you shocked me." I think he was angry that I had so painfully taken him away from his dream.

I don't remember what I said. Whatever it was, he seemed quickly to understand what we were doing. We finished getting his meds started, I paged the cardiologist, and within a half hour or so we had gone off for a catheterization and then to the coronary care unit. In a few days, the paddle burns had faded like a sunburn and he was doing well.

But I do remember that after we were finished, and until the time he went upstairs, one by one, the nurses who had been helping me all found reasons to slip back into his room for a brief conversation.

I didn't. So I never found out what else he may have remembered about his brief visit to the land of beautiful colors.

CHAPTER TEN

Now and Then It's Fun

F ROM TIME TO time I have been asked what it is, among all the things we do in the ER, that I find most enjoyable. Usually they expect something exciting, like intubation, or trauma resuscitations, or making a difficult diagnosis correctly. And it's true that those things, when they turn out well, are very satisfying.

But the correct answer is: none of these. I must confess that, for me, the task that is most fun—by which I mean that mixture of satisfaction, enjoyment, the sense of doing a skilled task well, and, yes, astounding and amazing the crowd—is, without question, fixing nursemaid's elbow.

Is . . . what?

The technical term for the problem is subluxation of the radial head. It happens in children from approximately age two up to age five or so, though I have seen it once in a seven-year-old. While it can occur in any kind of forceful play, it commonly happens when a child is walking with a parent—or with, as among the wealthy, a "nursemaid," hence the name. The adult is holding the child's hand as they walk, and when they reach a curb or a stair, the adult may pull upward on the child's arm, to assist them up to the next level. This means that the child's arm will first be fully outstretched and then pulled with enough force to lift the child off the ground. This kind of force, applied in this manner, is often sufficient to produce the injury.

The injury itself is a simple one. However, to understand it we need to go over some anatomy. There are three bones in the arm. The upper arm has one bone, the humerus. The forearm has two: the radius, which runs from the elbow to the wrist on the thumb side; and the ulna, which runs on the pinkie side. The ulna connects to the humerus via a large, hook-shaped joint that is very strong, but like a hinge, it permits the forearm to perform only two types of movements— flexion, that is, bending; and extension, that is, straightening.

Rotation of the forearm depends upon the joint between the radius and the humerus. This joint is not a hinge. Instead, the "head" of the radius (the elbow end) forms a shallow circular cup that fits neatly into a ball-shaped part of the end of the humerus. This permits limited motion but in all directions.

You can feel this very easily on yourself. Put your left hand under your right forearm by the elbow, and then flex your right forearm up and down. Your left hand can feel the ulna moving easily up and down as if hinged to the end of the humerus. Then, instead of flexing your forearm up and down, rotate it as if you are turning a screwdriver. Notice that now your ulna doesn't move at all. However, if you then put your left hand over your radius, you can feel it sliding back and forth over the ulna to produce that rotation. It's pretty nifty. You get stability from the ulna and flexibility from the radius.

Which brings us back to nursemaid's elbow. What happens is not actually a dislocation of the joint. Dislocations usually involve torn tissues, which require time to heal, if not actual surgical repair. However, with nursemaid's elbow, because the pull is in line with the length of the bone, there is no torsion to tear the joint. Instead, the head of the radius is simply tugged a little way out of its socket, without any real injury.

However, that "little way" is enough for the end of the bone to snag a bit of the ligament, like a bit of fabric getting stuck in a zipper. This is called subluxation. The joint is perfectly stable and everything is intact, but until that little bit of ligament is gotten out of the way, the child can't rotate or flex their forearm, and trying to do so hurts.

But now the injury has occurred, and you are the unfortunate parent, or older brother, or nursemaid. What do you think happened? You have just pulled hard on your child's arm, heard the child scream, and perhaps heard or felt a little popping sensation—and now your child is crying, their arm is dangling uselessly by their side, and when you try to move it, your child cries even harder. Is it any wonder that your next move is to jump in the car and drive at a dangerous speed to the nearest emergency room, all the while cursing yourself as a negligent caretaker?

That's the first part of why emergency physicians like this problem: it's a sudden traumatic injury that looks bad—and involves a child. The second part is that this is an injury we can fix. It's dead easy. It's quick. It's a complete cure. And parents can be completely reassured that they are good parents—except for the reckless driving. It's Dr. Feelgood all around.

So, a story.

I must begin with a disclaimer: If you ask my friends about me, what I am like, or who I remind them of, the name Clint Eastwood or John Travolta will not come up. In high school, I was terrible at sports. I received my athletic letter—which I never wore—in soccer. However, it was not for actually *playing* soccer, at which I was abysmal, but for being the manager of the team. In college, while I liked to think that my appearance was acceptable, most of my dating life involved falling in love with women who soon thereafter fell in love with someone else. Even at my present age, when I dance, I often find myself looking at my feet and repeatedly counting to two. It was pure blind luck that, in my late twenties, I met a wonderful woman who didn't seem to care about these deficiencies, and so for the last forty-five years I have been able to relax.

But now it is the mideighties. It's early afternoon. I am standing at the nurses' station, writing on a chart, when about twenty feet to my right, the ER door abruptly bursts open and a man comes stumbling in, holding a young boy. And as he comes through the door, the man is crying, "Help me. I think I broke his arm."

Without putting down my chart, I turn my head and look at the two of them. Instantly a few things are obvious. First, the boy is alert, looking around, and is not crying. He does not even look particularly upset. Second, while he is holding on to his father's shoulder with his right arm, his left arm is hanging down straight.

This is an important sign. When the elbow is broken or torn

internally, the bones bleed into the ball of connective tissue that seals the joint fluid within the joint. Hence, the bleeding puts pressure on the joint, and that hurts a lot. Straightening the arm out compresses the blood and joint fluid, which makes it hurt even more. Therefore, patients with a serious injury within the elbow joint will almost always hold their arm bent at ninety degrees, as if it were in a sling. Even with forearm injuries that don't involve the elbow, the swelling and pain are improved when you elevate the part that hurts.

But this boy's arm is hanging straight down. So I relax. (I don't normally relax when children are carried by their crying parents into the ER. No one does.) However, even in that first moment, I am 90 percent sure that whatever the boy's injury is, it is probably not very painful, that it is not an elbow fracture, and indeed—if the history checks out—probably not a fracture at all. That's not because I am particularly clever. It's simply that I have seen this before. Many times.

All this takes only a second or two to process. Raising a hand, I beckon the man to come directly over to me. The triage nurse who is in front of me has also witnessed his entry, and she nods: *I get it; you handle it for now.* Still holding the child, the man comes quickly to where I am standing.

The child seems to be about three or four years old. He looks a little apprehensive, but is still letting his arm dangle downward without seeming very uncomfortable.

I put down my pen and turn to face them both. "What happened?" I ask.

"I . . . we were playing in the yard . . . he was running by me, and I grabbed him by his arm. I was going to swing him, but . . . there was a cracking sound and he screamed and now he can't move his arm . . . I think I broke it." He seems close to tears.

"Let me see," I say.

I look at the boy, now speaking softly, telling him what I am doing as I do it. First, I hold his left hand in mine, and with my right hand I check his pulses. They are strong: I don't have to worry about any blood vessel problem right now. Not a surprise. Then I move upward, gently compressing the bones, looking for tenderness. I skip his elbow—if you think something is going to be painful to touch, save it for last—and move up his upper arm to his shoulder. Then I stabilize his forearm with my left hand and gently move his shoulder joint just a little in every direction. So far there is no evidence of pain.

Then I trade hands, now holding his left hand with my right, and with my left hand I gently palpate both sides of his elbow. He remains quiet while I do. But then, with my thumb, I press the upper part of his forearm just above the head of the radius. He flinches a little. "Is that where it hurts?" I ask. He nods quickly.

Last of all, still holding his elbow in my left hand, I gently lift his forearm at the wrist with my right hand, trying to flex his elbow. That hurts too. He wants to keep it straight and he doesn't want me to turn it.

All this has taken maybe four or five seconds.

"Okay," I say. (I am speaking directly to the boy. I always talk to children I am examining, no matter what their age.

Who knows what they understand?) "I'm going to move your arm now. It will hurt for a second. Then it will be better."

My left thumb is still over his radial head, pressing just enough that I can feel it beneath the skin. In my right hand, I am holding his left hand. His palm is facing mostly downward. Then, in four quick motions, I first rotate his palm downward some more till I meet a little resistance; then I flex his forearm upward until it almost touches his shoulder; and last, I rotate his forearm so his palm is now facing upward to the point of resistance; and then, equally firmly, I push his forearm back down again until it is once more fully extended, this time palm up. The boy cries out sharply, and at the same time I feel a little click under my left thumb—the feeling of the ligament slipping out of its trap. The whole maneuver takes only a second or two.

The father is looking at me, astonished, with the beginning of anger in his face: I pushed on his child's broken arm, making him cry in pain.

"Good," I say. "It's fixed now. Why don't you take him over to the waiting area"—I point with the clicky end of my pen—"and let him play for a bit until you are sure he is okay."

Now he is staring at his son, who, for the first time since the injury, spontaneously lifts his left hand up toward his face and looks at it.

The expression on the father's face says everything: complete amazement; the beginnings of indescribable relief. And—dare I say it—even a little awe.

I am relaxed and calm. I am Clark Kent; I am Robin Hood,

splitting the arrow at the Nottingham archery contest; I am Zorro; I am Walter Mitty on his best day; I am James Bond.

He stutters a thank-you, still watching his child now freely moving his arm. Then he starts to turn away.

"Oh, just one more thing," I say. He looks back at me questioningly.

"Before you go, you need to register him to be seen in the ER." I shrug. "It's one of the rules."

I twirl my twin pearl-handled Colt .45s, drop them into their holsters, and go back to writing on my chart.

Maybe when I get off shift tonight, Linda and I will go dancing.

CHAPTER ELEVEN

Riley

H E H A D A first name, but for the entire time I knew him, I called him Mr. Riley and he called me Dr. Seward. Most of our conversations were on the phone and in the context of prescriptions for ER patients. And in the ER, when we talked about him among ourselves, he was just "Riley."

Riley was the owner and principal pharmacist of Riley's Drugs, a pharmacy a few blocks from the hospital. This was the late eighties, and the large pharmacy chains were starting to come to town to compete with the mom-and-pop pharmacies that had been there for years. Despite the competition, Riley was a favored vendor both for people in the neighborhood and for the local emergency departments in that part of town.

There were a lot of reasons for this: he had been around for a long time; he was a well-known member of the community; and he was known to deal fairly with the less well-to-do clientele who lived in the neighborhood. But beyond all that, there was one big reason we all used him: Riley's was open until midnight.

This was not true of the chains—at least then. During the day, they were there for you, full service, shiny floors, bright lights, and well-stocked shelves. But when the sun went down, the lights turned off and they went home.

That system didn't work for the ER. We were not licensed to dispense medications, and evening was when things got busy. Evening was when the waiting room began to fill with coughing children whose mothers thought they felt warm; with asthmatics, whose breathing was starting to worsen; with people who had fallen and hurt themselves; with the elderly, who were having vague chest and abdominal pains that they hoped was just a little gas. Sometimes it was.

A lot of those people had had their symptoms for much of the day, hoping whatever it was would go away. But as the light grew dim, as the fevers went up and the breathing grew worse, they would finally get themselves into a car and come to the hospital. In those days—and since then as well—I thought of those people as the ER's—and Riley's—special responsibility.

By that I don't just mean Riley's Pharmacy; I mean Riley. Yes, he had other pharmacists who worked for him, and yes, I am sure he did go home some nights. But most of the time, after the sun went down, if someone needed an antibiotic, or a refill on their asthma inhaler, and if I picked up a phone to call it in, it was Riley I would be talking to.

So one day, after a couple of years of phone conversations, I decided that I wanted to meet him face-to-face. It was easy to arrange. After all, I was not only a doctor; I was a patient. I was in my midforties then, and like many of my own patients, I had some cholesterol problems and a touch of high blood pressure, and I too had prescriptions that needed to be filled. I don't remember what pharmacy I had been using. But I do remember that one night, after the customary couple of calls to Riley, I realized that I needed some way to tell him that what he was doing mattered. So a few days later, after working the seven-to-three shift, I drove over to his pharmacy, walked in with my prescriptions in hand, and said hello.

At first it felt a little strange. For one thing, he didn't look anything like my image of a pharmacist, and I don't think I looked too much like many of the physicians he was used to. I was after all a refugee from the sixties. My hair was long, I had a full beard, and when I talked I sounded like I was from California.

Riley reminded me of the sort of old man you might see in rural America, sitting on his front porch in bib overalls, overweight, smoking a cigar, and telling stories. That day he wasn't smoking a cigar, but he was probably smoking a cigarette. He was a chain smoker, and this was well before the days in which smoking cigarettes was banned in stores and health facilities. Riley sold them, and he smoked them as he did so. That was who Riley was.

This did not mean he was unprofessional. On the contrary. While his store was old, it was clean, it was organized, and it had all the things that patients needed. And that was also who Riley was.

We shook hands, I gave him my prescriptions, and we talked for a bit while he filled them for me. We got along immediately. We talked about family; and we talked about patients.

We both took care of the same people after all: those who came to the ER for much of their care, and who did so mostly at night. This generally meant that they were poor. And we both knew that these people were hardworking and honest, loved their families, and served their communities. In short, we had nothing in common, except that we both thought that taking care of people who didn't have much money was a good thing to do.

So after that first meeting, every couple of months, as my prescriptions needed refilling, I would stop by and say hello for a few minutes and chat, becoming gradually more comfortable in our conversation. One day I asked him whether he had ever been robbed. After all, his store was open till midnight, he was almost always alone there, and there certainly must be money in his cash drawer. Wasn't he scared?

I remember his smile, calm and unafraid. "No," he said. "I keep this." Then he reached under the counter, took out a short-barreled rifle, and showed it to me—not to touch, just to look at. I didn't ask him anything else. I just nodded at it and said something useless like "Well, I see what you mean." He put it back under the counter, we chatted a bit more as he finished my prescriptions, and then I left.

I didn't think that much about it. At that time, it was common to have a weapon in an establishment frequented by the public. Also, while our friendship was real, it was still a workplace friendship. Finally, despite years in the ER seeing what people can do to one another, I still didn't expect that sort of violent encounter to happen to anyone I knew personally. So I was surprised one day a year or so later when I came to work to hear everyone talking about what had happened at Riley's the night before.

It had evidently been around nine or ten o'clock. He was, as usual, alone in the store. A young man, perhaps in his late twenties, had come in and at first had just wandered about, looking at items on the shelves. Then, presumably when he was sure that there were no other customers, he came over to the prescription drop-off area. Riley went to assist him. But when he asked the young man what he needed, the man took out not a sheaf of prescriptions but a revolver. He pointed it at Riley and told him to give him all the cash.

I don't know precisely what happened next—whether Riley went to the cash register and pretended to be getting out the money, or whether he just reached under the counter. I do know that he came up with his gun, pointed it at the man's chest, and pulled the trigger. The man dropped to the floor and did not move again. Then Riley called the police.

They came immediately, called the coroner to deal with the body, and took Riley's statement about what had happened. I talked to the coroner later, and he said that Riley's aim had been good and the wound was through the heart. It was his opinion that the man had died nearly instantly. I don't think the police even took Riley down to the station, or if they did, they let him go home later that night. When the dust and paperwork had settled, the shooting was ruled self-defense and a justifiable homicide. And from a legal point of view, that was that.

In the ER, the general feeling was one of shock. But at the same time, we all felt that Riley had done the right thing.

He had defended himself, perhaps even saved his own life. Certainly he had made sure that no one would try to rob him again. If anything, Riley's stock in the ER had gone up. On the one hand, there were no high fives. But at the same time, we had all seen seriously wounded and dead people come to the ER after a robbery, and the fact that in this case the victim was the robber was okay with us.

Riley was not in the store the next day or the next. But within a week or so, he was back at work as usual, although I think that at first—perhaps permanently—he stopped working nights. I do know that a couple of weeks later I realized that I had not spoken to him, so I went over one afternoon just to say hello and find out how he was doing.

When I entered the store, even from across the room, I could see that something was wrong. He did not smile or greet me. He just looked up at me and nodded, obviously tired.

I asked him how he was. He didn't answer for a moment. Then he said, "I can't sleep."

I thought I knew what he meant.

"But you are safe now. Nobody's going to try to rob you again," I said.

He nodded. He continued to look at the counter. Even so, I could see that his eyes were red. Whether from sleeplessness or tears I couldn't tell. He went on as if I had not replied. "He comes to me when I dream," he said.

And suddenly I understood.

I said nothing. I did not know what to say.

Riley shook his head, still looking at the counter. Then he went on quietly. "He was so young."

He paused. Then he looked at me. "He didn't know what he was doing. He had a life in front of him, and I took it away." He said it as if he were reading it from a newspaper, with no emotion, only a deep fatigue that hinted at a hidden reservoir of pain. "I'm sure that's why he comes," he said.

For a little while we both were silent. Then I tried again.

"But if you hadn't shot him he might have killed you," I said.

He shrugged slightly. "Maybe. I don't know. Maybe not." His eyes were closed now, and he continued to shake his head. "But I *did* kill him. Now I can't stop thinking about him."

I didn't know how to respond. So I responded as a doctor. "Are you seeing someone about this?"

His eyes opened, and he thought about the question for a moment. Then he said something about how the pastor from their church came to talk to him. "But that doesn't change what I did," he said.

We both were silent, he sitting in his chair behind the counter, I standing on my side at the place where I would normally hand him prescriptions.

I thought about what he was trying to say. Then suddenly, as if some thoughtful stranger had handed me a note, I found myself asking, "When he comes to you, does he talk to you?"

Riley looked up at me, surprised. He thought about it. "No," he said, "he just comes. I don't think he has ever said anything."

"Do you know why he is coming? Do you think he wants anything from you?"

His answer was uncertain. "I don't know," he said.

I suddenly felt like I was treading water in the middle of a deep ocean, knowing nothing of what swam beneath me. All I knew for sure was that the good man sitting in front of me was in hell, and I did not know how to help him. At the same time, I felt as if I were right about something: whatever was going on in Riley's heart, it seemed to me that forgiveness was the key.

So after a moment I said, "The next time he comes, why don't you ask him what he wants?"

He looked back at me, frowned, and nodded just slightly.

I went on, "Maybe he just wants you to apologize. Maybe he wants to forgive you. But you have to ask."

Something worked. Around then he took a deep breath and reached over on the shelf for my small bag of prescriptions. "Thank you," he said.

I did not see him for several months after that. I heard that he had been taking a lot of time off, and other pharmacists were working his shifts. But one day when I came into work, the doctor I was relieving told me that Riley was in the hospital. He had had a small heart attack and was in some congestive failure.

So on my lunch break, I went up to his room and knocked on the door. He was sitting in bed, and in chairs around him were several members of his family—I believe his wife and I think a grown child or two, but I can't be sure. I know that he introduced me around, saying a couple of nice things. They all said hello. Then when I turned to Riley, they politely started talking again among themselves.

I remember very little of our conversation. I know that it

was not a long one. I know that I asked him whether he had talked to the man in his dreams. And I remember that he nodded at me, without smiling.

I asked him what he had said to the man. "I did apologize," he said, "but I don't think he said anything back. I'm not sure." He paused and then said, "He doesn't come by much anymore."

I did not know what to say. I shook his hand and told him to take it easy and get well, and then I went back to the ER.

I never saw him again. A few months later I heard that he had had another heart attack at home, and this one he did not survive. I think he was already in the process of selling the pharmacy, but certainly after his death the building was sold and I think did not open again. By then we had started a system of giving small medication starter packs to patients if the pharmacies were closed, and life went on.

Except for the young man who had come to his store with a gun. And except, of course, for Riley.

CHAPTER TWELVE

An Assault

I T IS NOT unusual for friends to ask me what a career in health care is like. When they do, they often say something to the effect of "I couldn't get used to the blood and gore." My usual answer is that the problem is not that it's hard to get used to blood and gore; the problem is that it's easy.

After all, we aren't the ones who are bleeding; we aren't the ones in pain. And we tend to get accustomed to things we see and do every day. As such, it is amazing how fast an injured human being, whose life has suddenly been torn apart, and who is in the midst of terrible pain and fear, can become "the motor vehicle crash in room six."

That's not necessarily a bad thing. After all, for a patient who has been injured, our first job is not to be tenderhearted; it is to save his life. That may mean such things as cutting a hole between his ribs and putting in a tube to drain the blood that is filling his chest.

But that doesn't mean we can't care about a patient as a human being. On the contrary, we must do so. And we must do so at the same time as we treat the object that is their body. So we move back and forth, from human interactions to acting on the object that is a particular human's body. And sometimes it is not easy to shift gears.

Which brings me to the only time I was ever physically assaulted by a patient.

He was a very old man, and sick, who had already begun the slow process of dying. He had been sent in from a nursing home because he had been eating poorly and getting increasingly lethargic. In such patients that usually means an infection.

He was not even officially my patient.

The doctor who had been taking care of him had come to the end of his shift. So he signed him over to me and went home. It was a simple sign-out: a comatose old man, getting some IV antibiotics for a kidney infection, waiting to go upstairs. No problem. Also, for the moment, there were no new charts in the rack. I was free. So I did a walk around.

I started with what I already thought of as the elderly coma. He was in a small four-bed ward, just behind the nurses' station. The nurse responsible for him was busy starting an IV on another patient, so I said hi and asked whether there was something I could do to help. (I am forever in debt to nurses. They have helped me beyond anything I could ever offer.)

"Really?" she said. I nodded.

"Well, the old guy in bed four needs a Foley. If you have time, would you mind putting it in?"

Sure, I said. Why not?

A Foley catheter is a simple device. It's just a rubber tube with a small doughnut-shaped balloon at the end. There is a much smaller tube running along the length of the catheter from the balloon to the outside world, through which it can be inflated. The catheter is designed to be inserted through the urethra into the bladder. Then the balloon is inflated, preventing the catheter from sliding back out. Urine can then drain out passively through the tube into a container where it can be measured accurately. Formerly it was also used as a convenience in the management of patients who were bedridden. However, because it can lead to infections in the bladder, this practice is now much less common.

Inserting a Foley catheter is generally not difficult. You clean the area, and then, using sterile gloves, you lubricate the tube with K-Y Jelly and slide it into the patient's urethra and up into the bladder. Then you inflate the balloon with water so that, in theory, the end cannot slide back out, and attach a collection tube to the other end.

Nurses usually are the ones who do it, but it is a procedure that emergency physicians also need to know how to do well, so a little practice never hurts.

The kit was already set up by the right side of the bed, and the patient was as advertised: very old, emaciated, and comatose. He was breathing regularly with good color but did not rouse in the slightest when I listened to his chest, felt his abdomen, and checked his pupils.

Therefore, after removing his diaper, I put on my sterile gloves and took his penis in my left hand. I held it upward while I painted the end liberally with an antiseptic solution. Next, with my right hand, which was still sterile, I grasped the Foley near the end, rubbed the tip in a generous pile of lubricating jelly, and introduced it into the urethra. When I did so, the patient stirred lightly but did not open his eyes. So I continued sliding the Foley further through his urethra.

A comment at this point: putting in a Foley is a significantly different procedure in a man than it is in a woman. I cannot say which sex has more discomfort from the procedure, but in men, there is one very important obstacle: the prostate gland. In younger men, this is about the general size and shape of a marshmallow, though substantially firmer. It completely surrounds the urethra, something like an olive on a toothpick. It has several functions, but chief among them is providing some constituents for the seminal fluid that help keep the sperm alive at the time of intercourse. In addition, prostates have an annoying habit of occasionally developing cancer.

But most important, as men get older, their prostates get bigger. This is not a problem in terms of their outer diameter. However, their inner diameter—that is, the passageway through which urine must flow—gets accordingly smaller. This is the reason for the near universal complaint of older men that they have trouble passing urine.

But that enlargement makes it hard not only for urine to come out but for Foley catheters to go in. This gentleman was no exception.

This is normally not a great problem. One simply moves the penis around in various directions with the left hand while continuing to exert some pressure with the right. However, by then things are often a bit slippery, and you need to be careful not to lose your grip on either the penis or the Foley.

(Do I sense that some of you out there have found another reason to forgo a career in medicine?)

And I was paying attention. I was, in fact, bent over and concentrating deeply on the task at hand (as it were) and therefore did not notice that my "comatose" patient was waking up.

Until, out of the corner of my eye, I saw him slowly sit upright.

I was startled. Sitting up was not part of the description I had been given. I stood up and looked at him.

For a moment, he sat there, staring at me, saying nothing. Then—slowly, oh so slowly—he lifted his right arm, and—slowly, oh so slowly—swung it around in a gentle arc, until—slowly, oh so slowly—his fist landed on the side of my chin.

It did not hurt. It was more like a butterfly landing on a flower than a punch in the jaw.

But I was amazed. This elderly man, who I had been treating as if he were a simple mechanical problem of tubes, lubricants, and appropriate positioning, had awoken from a coma, sat up, and punched me in the face.

I did not move. He remained sitting for a moment, still staring at me. Then, without saying a word, he closed his eyes, lay back on the bed, and returned to his coma.

I stood there, not knowing how to respond. Then, still with his penis in one hand and the Foley in the other, I turned and looked at the nurse. She had been standing just beyond the next bed and had seen the whole thing. I think it was all she could do to keep from falling on the floor with laughter.

I asked her if she could help, so she came around the bed and held the patient's hands, both for comfort and for restraint, while I finished the procedure. Then she headed out to the front nurses' station to share the news of my assault.

When I tell this story, it usually gets some sort of a laugh. And I laugh too. But I think of that elderly man in a different way than I did when I first encountered him: not as emaciated, frail, and dying but how he must have been when he was young.

After all, once he had been young. Perhaps he had been in love. Perhaps he had children, and had sometimes tossed them in the air and caught them as they laughed. Perhaps he had worked hard at a job. Perhaps he had lived in a community of people whom he cared about and who cared about him.

All that may have disappeared, but the person who had done those things still lived inside that body and in that mind, even as they both faded away. Clearly he was still alive enough to be angered by some strange man who, without warning, had grabbed him in his private place and had hurt him for no reason he could understand. So he had responded as he would have when he was young, by fighting back.

In that moment, for me, he stopped being the elderly man in a coma and became the human being he had never ceased to be.

CHAPTER THIRTEEN

A Rash

I T WAS QUARTER to seven in the evening.

My shift was scheduled to end at seven. I had finished admitting or discharging all the patients I had been caring for, and I didn't really want to pick up another chart with so little time left. So I was helping one of the nurses push a patient on a gurney back from the X-ray department. As we went by the nurses' station, I looked up at the clock and realized that, amazingly enough, I was going to go home on time. Punctually at seven o'clock, I really would say good night to everyone and walk out the door. That hardly ever happened.

Now, I like to think of myself as someone who mostly likes his job, and is no more selfish than most people. Even so, I was just finishing a twelve-hour shift, and I confess that the thought that in fifteen minutes I was going to be walking out of the ER, into the warm Georgia evening and on my way home, made me smile.

The smile did not last long.

We continued past the nurses' station and started to cross the long hallway that ran through the entire ER, from the ambulance entrance to the doors that led to the rest of the hospital. As we did so, the doors to the ambulance bay swung open, admitting a gurney being pushed by two EMTs. It headed directly toward us, moving fast. As they approached, the lead EMT said loudly, to anyone who might be listening: "She was talking to us on the way in. But now she won't say anything. And she's breaking out in a rash." I turned my head and looked in the direction of the voice.

The back of the moving gurney was in the upright position, supporting a young woman, sitting up, who was mostly covered by a sheet. She was pale and ill-appearing, and looked around the room with a confused expression, as if she saw nothing that she could recognize. As she approached us, I could clearly see her face and one bare arm. Both were speckled with random red spots, not a lot of little ones like measles spots, but fewer and larger.

At that moment, in a single flash, I had several simultaneous thoughts, each with a sense of utter certainty.

The first was: *Oh, my God.*

The second was: *We need to get her treatment started right now.*

The third was: *But it's probably already too late. By sometime tomorrow she will probably be dead.*

Last of all was: *I guess I'm not going to be home on time after all.*

So much for unselfishness.

There was an empty critical care bay across the long hall from where I was standing. One of the nurses—I don't remember who—guided the EMTs there with the gurney. I also have no memory of grabbing a mask and putting on a gown and gloves, but I must have done so. What I do remember next was standing beside the gurney and beginning my examination, while two nurses rapidly started two IVs and drew several tubes of blood.

A comment on examining patients:

The history and the physical examination (H&P) are the heart and soul of medicine. They are how doctors think about patients. The "history" is what we learn by asking questions; the "physical" is what we learn by looking, touching, feeling, and listening to the sounds the body makes as it does its work. Between them, these two procedures are simple enough to be a common framework of knowledge for all physicians to use as they make records or communicate with one another, yet they are flexible enough to encompass literally any problem in any degree of complexity.

Therefore, depending on the situation, an H&P can take a long time, often up to an hour for a new patient in a private practice. Or it might be just a few minutes for a follow-up visit for a known problem. The framework is the same for both; it just depends on what is needed.

My initial history and physical on this young woman took under thirty seconds.

First I asked the EMT what he knew. His answer was that he had been called to the patient's home about forty-five minutes prior because she had developed a fever and was starting to act funny. The mother told him that she had been sick for only about a day with a sore throat, and had been in bed, taking Tylenol. However, an hour before, her fever had gone up to over 104 and she had started to become confused about where she was. She also complained of a headache. On his examination, she was responsive but confused, and appeared to be very ill, so they had put her in the ambulance and taken her to the ER as fast as possible.

While I listened to his story, I was also helping the nurse take off her pajama top and cover her with a sheet. Then I listened briefly to her heart and lungs and felt her abdomen for any signs of tenderness. At that point she wasn't answering questions, though she did squeeze both my hands with both of hers when asked. At the same time, I got a closer look at her rash.

It was, as I had thought, no ordinary rash. Her chest and abdomen, and to some extent her face and arms, showed randomly scattered petechiae and purpura throughout, and they had begun to appear on her legs as well.

Petechiae are small irregular red spots that are notable because when you push on them, they don't disappear. Rashes such as hives or measles are caused by a widening of the small blood vessels in the skin. They show up as small red dots or blotches. However, when you push on them, the blood is compressed forward into the veins so that, when you remove your finger, the blotch will have vanished—until a few seconds later, when the capillaries fill up again.

Petechiae are different. They are caused not by a dilation of the blood vessels but by the actual destruction of their walls, so that the blood leaks out into the surrounding tissue. When you push on such a blotch, the blood does not go away; there is no place for it to go. Purpura is the same thing except that the blotch is not just a small dot from a small vessel but a large patch of blood from a larger one—almost like a bruise.

Big or little, both mean the same thing: there is something going on in the body that does not simply irritate the blood vessels; it destroys them.

However, the local destruction of the blood vessels is not, by itself, the problem. The problem is the disease that is causing that destruction. For example, sometimes people can get petechiae on their face and upper chest just from coughing very hard and increasing the pressure in the local small vessels. They are real petechiae, but at bottom the problem is just a cough. Or sometimes petechiae can be caused by a problem with blood clotting. The blood vessels are indeed damaged, but medications that fix the clotting problem will stop the process.

The truly dangerous situation occurs when a localized infection—say, a sore throat or a skin infection—spreads from its local site into the bloodstream. Even this may not be immediately destructive. Some organisms that get in the bloodstream simply go somewhere else and cause other localized infections. This is still a dangerous situation, but there is time to make diagnoses and begin treatments. The disaster occurs when the organism that is released into the bloodstream is one that has the capacity to cause major destruction of the tissues it invades. In this case, once it is in the bloodstream, not only can it travel everywhere, it will also destroy whatever tissue the bloodstream takes it to.

Neisseria meningitidis is one such organism. And *Neisseria meningitidis* was what I was sure she had.

Surprisingly enough, colonization by *Neisseria*—having it in one's body without producing any disease—is common. In some studies, the number of normal people who have *Neisseria* growing in their throats is as high as 10 percent, without causing any seeming harm. Furthermore, such carriers are not usually the people who acquire the disease. Instead, for reasons that are still not clear, it seems to appear sporadically, presumably spread from someone who is a carrier to someone who is susceptible—and it is most frequently the susceptibles who get the disease.

This seems to occur most often in situations where adolescents and young adults are concentrated in groups, such as colleges and military bases. Typically, everyone will appear to be completely well, until suddenly, with no warning, some perfectly healthy individual will come down with a serious infection. When that happens, it is possible for a few other healthy people who have had a close exposure to the sick person also to acquire the disease, with equal suddenness. (It is for this reason that experts recommend that young people planning to go into the military or attend college be vaccinated against this organism.)

The infection can occur in two ways. Sometimes it is localized to the coverings of the brain (the meninges) and the spinal fluid. This, by itself, is a serious and often rapidly fatal disease. However, not infrequently the disease will spread throughout the entire body, damaging and destroying large areas, and usually killing the patient. Those who do survive may lose limbs, or internal organs, or be seriously disfigured.

For physicians who see sick patients, this is basic knowledge. That is why my thirty-second examination—sudden onset; adolescent; abrupt high fever; appearing seriously ill; petechiae and purpura recently appearing and spreading rapidly—was enough to tell any ER physician that her most urgent need was not further diagnosis but immediate treatment. At that point the IV was running, so I asked the nurse to bring me what she already knew I would want.

"She needs two grams of Rocephin IV push now."

"Connor is already drawing it up." I did not need to ask. Connor had been an ER nurse for years.

He was back in under a minute and immediately started pushing the medicine, a powerful antibiotic in a high dose that was very effective against the *Neisseria* bacteria.

I checked the time. It had been just under four minutes since she came through the door.

"Four minutes, door to drug. That's excellent work," I said. They both nodded quietly. No one was celebrating yet. At that point, I asked them to add a 500 mg IV of vancomycin over one hour—not the best antibiotic for this organism but one that does kill organisms that have become resistant to Rocephin.

The first nurse was rechecking vital signs. The patient had a rapid heart rate, about 120—what it would be if she were running easily. Her blood pressure was maintaining well at around 110/65, and with oxygen running through a nasal cannula, her blood oxygen saturation was 100 percent. Her rectal temp was 104, and she was breathing reasonably well at about eighteen times per minute. Even so, I knew she was likely already a little dehydrated just from the fever and being sick all day, so I asked the nurse to run in a liter of normal saline through her IV, then wrote orders for a blood count, electrolyte determination, blood cultures, and a lactic acid level to be done on the blood they had already drawn.

A more careful repeat examination added little to what I already knew. The only new finding was that when I examined the flexibility of her neck, it was normal.

Meningitis also affects the tissues surrounding the spinal cord, and a common sign of the disease is stiffness and pain in the neck. In her case, that she had none was not reassuring. You cannot have a war without both sides fighting; if you do not hear the sounds of battle, it usually means that the defenders have laid down their arms. In the same way, it was possible that the flexibility was not due to the absence of infection but the failure of her body to fight against it.

And if that was the case, there was nothing I could do to change it.

I asked who the ICU attending physician was that night.

The nurse looked over at a chalkboard just behind me. "Dr. Tristan," she said.

"Thank you," I said, and went back to the nurses' station to give him a call. He was at home and answered immediately. I told him the problem. He had only one question: "What about steroids?"

"She just got the Rocephin but I will give them now."

He said he would be in as soon as possible and would do the lumbar puncture (the spinal tap, to see whether she had meningitis as well). Then he hung up the phone. I told the nurse to give 10 mg IV of Decadron to the patient. I didn't think it would change things, but it was one of those medications for which the recommendations continue to change over time, I didn't think it could hurt, and I was ready to grasp at a straw.

At that moment, the patient representative came by. "Hi, Paul," she said, "I've got her mother and her sister in the quiet room; are you ready to talk to them?"

I put the phone down and looked at her. "Depends on what you mean by 'ready,' " I said without smiling.

"I know," she said, and gave me a quick pat on my hand. "Shall we go?"

I told the ward clerk that if Dr. Tristan came before I finished, he should tell him that I was talking to the family. The quiet room wasn't far, just around the corner of the hallway.

It's hard to give people bad news. At the same time, it is often the most important thing I do. What I had to tell them was that someone they loved had just contracted a very dangerous disease. Worse yet, on arrival, she was already far down the path. While they themselves might not yet have realized it, the people to whom I would be talking were almost certainly in the middle of the worst kind of family tragedy: the death of a child. In those situations, the most powerful emotion is grief; but the second-most-powerful emotion is rage.

It is impossible for family members not to second-guess

themselves, to look for things they did wrong—and for wrong things that other people might have done. Those are the kinds of questions that can tear families apart, and destroy the lives of people who were close to the person who has died. My patient might be dying, but her family was going to be around for a long time, and what I asked and what I said might make a difference—for better or for worse—in how they survived this disaster.

When we entered the quiet room, I found two women waiting there. One was the patient's mother, the other her sister. They were sitting together on the couch. I sat down in a chair across from them.

The first thing I did was introduce myself and shake their hands.

I asked if they needed anything. A glass of water? A cup of coffee? They shook their heads no.

Then I asked them what they understood about what was going on. I am often astounded at how different that understanding can be from what I take for granted. And that is especially true in matters of life and death. I was not surprised to hear that they really had no idea.

Then I asked them to go over what had happened: When had she gotten the initial sore throat? What had happened afterward? And what had made them want to take her to the hospital?

Again, it was not surprising. They hadn't thought much about her sore throat, and it was only the fever and that she wasn't feeling well that morning that had made her mother keep her home. She had noted that her daughter was feeling a little worse at noon and still had a fever, so she had given her a Tylenol. Then she told her to rest, but to call her if she felt worse. She did not hear from her daughter that afternoon, and she thought she was sleeping; therefore, she did not disturb her. It was only when her other daughter came home that they did check on her and discovered how much more ill she appeared.

Then it was my turn.

Many years earlier, when I was in my pediatric residency, I watched a hematologist inform the parents of a five-year-old boy that he had leukemia, and that, given our medical knowledge in those days, he was going to die. Then, for another hour, he talked to them about the "but" clauses: but right now, there were a lot of medicines that he could give him that would put him into remission; but remissions could sometimes last for a very long time; but we could not know what new medical discoveries might be made in the meantime; but he would do everything that could be done. But most of all, he would be there with them all the way.

He did not lie to them. He told the hard truth; and then he gave them all the hope there could possibly be.

I also began with the bad news. I told them that the patient had acquired an extremely dangerous and destructive infection. I told them the name—meningococcemia. I told them how rapidly it progressed, and that it was very destructive and often fatal. Also, I said that the disease had already progressed significantly and would be difficult to reverse.

However, I also said that we had already given her the medicine that was needed to kill the germ. What we had to do now was to see whether we had done so in time for the process of destruction to stop and reverse. I said that she would soon be going to the ICU, where they could continue doing what we were doing now: monitoring her vital signs, and supporting her blood pressure and breathing. By morning, we would know which way things would go.

They were quiet for a moment. Then the mother asked if I would talk to another daughter who lived about three hundred miles away. There was a phone in the room so she placed the call, talked to her daughter for a moment, and handed me the phone.

My conversation with her daughter was brief. Most of what I said was a repetition of what I had already said to the patient's mother. But then, at the end, she asked me a question that let me know that she too had not allowed herself to understand how serious things were. She asked, "Do you think I need to come?"

I thought for a moment. Then I said the only thing I knew with absolute certainty. "You know how, now and then, there are times when the family needs to be together?"

"Yes," she answered.

"Well," I said, "this is one of those times."

For a moment, she didn't say a word. Then she said, "I'll be there as soon as I can."

I gave the phone back to her mother and asked if she had more questions.

She shook her head.

Then I said, "In that case, there is one more thing I need to say to you both."

They looked at me silently.

I went on, "I don't know what is going to happen. But I do know one thing: whatever happens, it is not your fault."

They still said nothing, but they watched me closely, as if, should they look away, something important might be lost.

"You already know that this is a disease that comes on fast. But you may not realize just how fast. You see, when the disease was localized to a sore throat, she wasn't very sick. It was only when the bacteria burst into her bloodstream and spread everywhere throughout her body that she began to get sick enough for you to see that something unusual was happening.

"But more than just the speed of the disease, the thing that is going to make the difference is not just that the germs have gotten everywhere; after all, most of them have already been killed by the antibiotic. What matters now is whether the poisons that are being released into the bloodstream by the destroyed tissues—things that impair blood clotting, that damage the immune system—are already too plentiful and will continue to damage tissue and release more poisons. That can become a vicious cycle, one that there never was anything you could do about and for which even we can only provide support. At this point, what matters is whether her body is sufficiently intact to manage the damage that has already occurred, and fix itself."

I sat still for a moment. Then I said, "I know that sounds complicated. And it is. And you can forget everything I just said. But I do want you to remember one thing."

I paused. Then I spoke more slowly: "Remember this: no

matter what happens, it is not your fault." Then I repeated what I had said before. "No matter what happens, it is not your fault."

I waited for a second. Then I asked, "Is there anything else you would like to know?"

They both shook their heads no.

"Okay. I'm going back out to keep an eye on things. I will tell you when she goes to the ICU."

When I went back out, Dr. Tristan had already arrived. The young woman was still stable, but he was going to take her to the ICU and put in some monitoring lines. We talked a little about some other possible drug therapies, and then I took him back and introduced him to the family. I think by the time all the loose ends were tied up and I had finished my charting, it was nearly nine. So I went home.

She died about ten o'clock the following morning. Her sister had arrived in time to be with the family when she died.

CHAPTER FOURTEEN

To Breathe

THE CHART DID not seem particularly exciting: a forty-two-year-old male seeking help for alcoholism.

It's a common complaint. While most treatment programs' staff can manage the detox—the process of waiting for the alcohol to wear off—they may not be able to manage other unrelated medical problems. Therefore, before they will accept a patient, they require a medical evaluation. As many people with alcohol problems do not have a physician, they often take care of this by coming to the ER.

This patient did not fit the stereotype of the disheveled and unshaven alcoholic. He was a pleasant gentleman in early middle age: well dressed, clean shaven, and looking rather prosperous. He did not even seem particularly intoxicated.

I was not surprised. A serious alcoholic who has been drinking steadily for a while can have astounding amounts of alcohol on board and still seem reasonably sober.

I began by introducing myself and asking about his need for treatment: How long had he had a problem with alcohol? When was his last drink? What other medications did he take? Was he allergic to anything? And what made him decide to come in for treatment at this particular time? It turned out that, though he had been drinking heavily and steadily for a few weeks, he had not had a drink in the last two days. As to his reason for coming in that day, it seemed to be a combination of becoming personally more frightened about how out of control his drinking was, and the fact that he had begun to feel increasingly unwell.

I could see that. His hands were trembling, and he seemed anxious and uncomfortable. I asked him whether he would like something to help those symptoms, and he promptly agreed. He already had an IV in place—the triage nurse had noted his tremors and anticipated the possible need—so I asked the nurse who was assisting me to give him a 4 mg IV of Ativan. It's in the family of benzodiazepines, and is particularly effective in alcohol withdrawal. Usually it works just fine.

Usually.

At first it seemed to help. He became significantly calmer, his tremors eased, and I was able to continue. However, I was only about halfway through the physical examination when things stopped being routine. First, quite abruptly, he again started to become more anxious. His hands started shaking again. Most alarming of all, he began to sweat. We have already discussed how sweating with no obvious cause is a sign of danger. I recommended another four milligrams of Ativan and again he readily agreed.

This time, though, the effect was not so impressive. When he was admitted to the ER, his vital signs—pulse, blood pressure, respiratory rate, and temperature—had all been normal. However, on rechecking, his pulse was now between 110 and 120 beats per minute and his pressure was 160/90—not only high but rising.

I asked the nurse to put him on the monitor. By that time, he was sweating enough that the nurse had to dry his chest with a towel to get the leads to stick. The monitor confirmed my reading of his vital signs and continued to track them. About then he asked if he could have some more medicine. I was happy to oblige. This time I gave him eight milligrams.

To put this in perspective, the average person who uses Ativan now and then to treat anxiety may take somewhere between one-half and two milligrams and does so by taking a slowly absorbed pill form. My patient had just had roughly eight times that amount, given through an IV, which starts to work in the brain in under a minute. If, instead of his pill, that same average person took that much that quickly, he would be unconscious for hours and might even need some help in remembering to breathe. However, this gentleman was not only showing no signs of any sedation, he was getting worse. Most alarming was the fact that he was starting to become confused. In short, he was heading like a freight train straight into a bad case of delirium tremens.

I think everyone has heard of the D.T.'s. They turn up frequently in literature and cartoons in the form of people believing that bugs are crawling all over them or hallucinating pink elephants. What is not so widely known is that the D.T.'s are a true medical emergency. The danger is that D.T.'s affect not just the brain but the entire body, and as the agitation and delirium worsen, they can progress to severe and prolonged seizures that themselves are life-threatening. Even without seizures, the agitated delirium can cause the patient to injure himself. Finally, in the worst cases, the disease impairs the body's ability to regulate such vital functions as temperature, heartbeat, blood pressure, and even breathing. When such basic processes are out of control, death is not far behind.

I gave the Ativan one more try, but with bad D.T.'s, even a drug as strong as Ativan can be like spitting on a bonfire. I didn't expect much, and not much was what I got. He was now actively hallucinating and no longer understood my words. Furthermore, he was also trying to get off the gurney and required two nurses to keep him from doing so. At that point, I felt that there was only one thing left that I could do—something I had never previously needed to do for D.T.'s: I needed to put him down.

No, I don't mean that difficult thing you have the vet do to your beloved family dog when he or she becomes too old and sick to manage. Nor did I only want a good way to restrain him. What I needed to do was to take the agitated part of his brain offline, thereby shutting down all the activity that was causing his vital signs to go out of whack. Furthermore, I needed to do so in a manner that would allow me to keep his body functioning normally and safely until the storm calmed down.

The best way to do this is a procedure called rapid sequence intubation. Taking that phrase apart, it means a procedure in which, rapidly but with extreme care, we perform a sequence of tasks that result in the patient being profoundly sedated, but with a tube in his windpipe so that we can continue to breathe for him while he is too unconscious to do so himself.

We'd talked about this procedure before in the ER, whenever we discussed resuscitation. In fact, we'd talked about it so often that it probably seemed like it was no big deal: splint a sprained ankle, sew up a cut, put a tube in someone's windpipe. Now let's have lunch.

But in this situation, there was a difference: this patient was not already dead. In most of the situations in which we intubate patients in the ER, the patients are in extremis, and when a patient is already close to death, you may sometimes make things better, but it's difficult to make them worse.

But this gentleman was very much alive. In fact, if the Ativan had worked, he might have been able to walk to detox under his own power. But what I planned to do was take away all the reflexes and abilities he was currently using to breathe, and then, before he could suffocate, replace them with my own.

Doing that is a big deal, even if we do it so often it seems routine.

In this sense, it's like the routine big deal that airline pilots do. Let's say we want to hop a plane to Miami. So we go down to the airport, buy our ticket, and find our seat. Then the pilot starts the engines, opens the throttle, pulls back on the wheel, and up we go. At the other end, the pilot puts the nose down, lands on the runway, and taxis to where we get out, and—poof—we are in Miami. It's routine, and happens that way every time.

Almost.

Those extremely rare times when it doesn't go right, when it's not routine, are the times when we have a small sense of what an incredible miracle it is that pilots and those who work in commercial air travel perform every day.

Endotracheal intubation is also routine. And it really does go well almost every time. You need have no more fear of it than you do of getting on an airplane. Even so, like flying in an airplane, it is routine and successful not because it is easy; it isn't. Putting a plastic tube through someone's mouth, down their throat, and into their windpipe is doing something that the body is not remotely designed to tolerate, and which requires a great deal of anatomical and pharmacologic ingenuity to accomplish. Also, of all the procedures we do in the ER, endotracheal intubation is the one that we least want to do wrong.

You have seen an ET tube. It's the skinny plastic thing sticking out of someone's mouth on TV shows when the actor is supposed to be in the hospital in a coma. If you were to take the tube out of his mouth and examine it, you would see that it had some holes along its barrel, some numbered lines on the outside so that the person managing the tube knows how far in it is, and a bulb at the tip that, once it has gone down past the vocal cords and into the trachea, can be filled with air to keep the oxygen from leaking out when it is pushed into the lungs. All we need to do is put the tube in correctly. But doing so is where the problem comes in.

You see, for an intubated patient, the tube is not merely one source of oxygen to breathe—it is the only source. Therefore, if by some chance the tube does not go into the trachea and instead goes down the esophagus, the patient ceases to get any oxygen at all. It doesn't matter why he needed to be intubated, or even whether it was necessary at all. If we put the tube into the esophagus, then we will be blowing the oxygen into his stomach instead of his lungs. If we do not recognize that fact and fix it immediately, the patient will die.

But how is putting the tube in the wrong place even possible?

It's possible because the construction of our respiratory tract represents one of nature's great practical jokes.

The problem is that oxygen is not only an essential nutrient: it is one we cannot do without for more than a few minutes. Effective breathing cannot be put on hold. Even so, for some strange reason, nature has arranged things so that, when humans breathe, they do so through the same hole through which they eat and drink. However, if food and water get into our lungs, they can gum them up completely and we will die. This means that every time we take a drink of water or eat a bite of food, our breathing system must shut itself down and completely seal itself off, until the food or drink goes by.

This is an arrangement that makes no sense whatsoever. It is as if, in a busy airport, the single major runway for all takeoffs and landings runs across the most crowded street in the city, and all that busy traffic now and then has to stop to let the arriving and departing flights go by. (This is actually the case for the airport in Gibraltar, the British territory at the entrance to the Mediterranean Sea, where the famous rock is located. Fortunately, it does not have a lot of flights.)

But there is another problem, even more dangerous than simply having to shut down and then restart our breathing mechanism several hundred times a day. Everything that enters our throat—air or food—has two possible destinations: the lungs or the stomach. This means that our throat not only has to constantly switch the tracks, it must choose the right track for the right nutrient—air for the lungs, food and water for the stomach—and it must be absolutely correct, every single time.

The amazing thing is that we do both these things very well. We make the correct decision about which goes where; and then we completely and successfully either seal off or reopen our trachea whenever it is necessary to do so. We accomplish this miracle through an extremely complex and almost completely automatic trick that we do many times each day. We call it swallowing.

Here's how it works. So long as we aren't eating or drinking anything, then your tongue and the muscles in our throat position themselves so that nothing solid or liquid in our mouth—even saliva—will go any further. During that time, our trachea is wide open. We can breathe, we can sing, we can talk or whistle or perform all our other daily oral chores.

But when we choose to swallow, everything reverses. First, a little trapdoor just above our trachea, called the epiglottis, slams down on the tracheal opening and seals it off completely. As it does so, our tongue and the muscles in our pharynx (the back part of the mouth) push the food or water into the top part of our throat. Then rings of muscle contract in sequence, one after another, passing the food or water from squeeze to squeeze, all the way down to our stomach. Only after the food or drink has completely gone by and the danger has passed does the epiglottis open again to let the air in. And it does that correctly every time.

There you have it: an incredibly stupid anatomical flaw is patched by a truly miraculous switching system.

But what does this have to do with putting in an endotracheal tube?

Think of the endotracheal tube as being a special kind of food. It also enters through the mouth. Therefore, it faces all the obstacles of anatomy and muscle reflexes that are designed to prevent things in the mouth from going into the windpipe. Those obstacles are not small. If you were to take a spoon, put it in your mouth, and start to push it toward the back of your throat, you would immediately discover just how hard your body will resist your doing so. (I do not recommend that you try this experiment; you already know how it will turn out. And I don't want anyone out there choking themselves by accident.)

But reflexes aren't the only problem. An ET tube is both long and hard, and in addition to bypassing muscle reflexes, it must also make its way around a very substantial blind curve. For a normal human, facing forward, the tunnel from the lips to the windpipe requires a turn of well over ninety degrees, from backward to downward and then slightly forward. So how do we get our ET tube past these obstacles of muscular response, curvature, and anatomy? How can we even see the way to go?

Normally, we can't. Therefore, in order to see where to pass the tube, we need to get rid of these obstacles.

The first thing that must go are all those muscular reflexes in our tongue, palate, and throat. That means that the patient not only must be put into a profound sleep, he must be completely paralyzed to prevent even unconscious protective reflexes from operating.

Then, once the muscles are relaxed, the curve in the passageway made by the mouth, throat, and windpipe must be straightened out, to see where the tube is supposed to go. We do this via a very precise series of maneuvers. First, we tip the head upward. This straightens out the first part of the curve. Then the whole head, still tipped upward, must move forward as a unit; this straightens out the second part of the curve. If maneuvers are done correctly with anatomy that permits it, then at that point you have a passageway through which you can see the opening of the trachea.

That is, you could see it if you got the intervening floppy anatomy out of the way: the tongue and the epiglottis.

For this we use a special tool called a laryngoscope. This is basically a long, thin metal blade, either straight or with an upward curve, that has a small light at its tip. (It's called a "blade" but it is too dull to cut anything.) Attached to the back end is a handle that sticks upward at ninety degrees. When held correctly it looks like a small upside-down pickax.

Standing at the head of the patient, which is now tipped back, facing you, and upside down, you hold the laryngoscope in your left hand—right- and left-handed people use the same scope, always in the left hand—slide the blade into the patient's mouth, and then use it to shove the tongue, which is now on top and hanging down, toward the left, out of the way. Next, without losing control of the tongue, you continue to slide the blade down the throat until you come to the epi-glottis, and with the tip of the blade, you lift it up and out of the way. Now, if all has gone well, you can actually see the opening of the trachea and the vocal cords beyond. If so, without ever looking away from those beautiful vocal cords, you take the endotracheal tube in your right hand and slide it past the right side of the blade, between the vocal cords, and into the trachea.

You are still not finished. You must be sure that the tube has gone far enough into the trachea that the bulb at the end is below the cords and can be inflated without damaging them. But you must be equally sure that the tube has not gone so far that it has passed the place where the trachea divides into the two bronchial tubes, entering one of them and there-fore blocking air from entering the other. Only when you are certain of all that can you inflate the bulb, so its sides press against the wall, making sure that the system doesn't leak and that the air can go in and out only through the tube.

Even then you aren't finished. Now comes the most critical part of the entire procedure: verifying that the tube is going to stay where it is supposed to be. Remember, even if the patient who has just been intubated could breathe by him-self before the tube went in, he can't do it anymore. All the things we had to do to make it possible for him to tolerate the tube—sedation, paralysis, and the intubation itself—now make it impossible for him to breathe or speak on his own. Therefore, if by some unfortunate chance, the intubator has put the tube in the wrong place, the patient can't tell you; you need to figure it out by yourself. And you must do so immediately and then continue to monitor it constantly, for as long as the tube is in place.

Does that sound difficult? Did your palms sweat a little as you imagined yourself doing the procedure? It is, and they should.

But here is the good news. First, there are lots of ways to make sure the tube is in the right place. Nowadays, there are probes inside the tube that will immediately—and continually—detect the presence of carbon dioxide in the exhaled air, something that will happen only if the tube is in the windpipe. There are also detection devices that we can put on the tube that change color when CO_2 passes through them. We constantly watch the patient's oxygen levels via an electronic clip on his finger. And there is the good old-fashioned way, which we used before all those tools were invented: you can examine the patient. You can listen to the lungs to see whether air is moving in and out, and then listen to the stomach to be sure that it is not.

All these things represent the paradox that is true of airplanes and intubation; they are both very safe, safer than riding a bicycle on the street, going swimming in the ocean, or climbing a ladder—activities that even children can do. But they are safe, in spite of their intrinsic difficulty, because of all that has been done and continues to be done to make it so.

You need not be afraid of having to be intubated. We are afraid on your behalf. And as a result, the complications of failed airway management are rare—certainly much more rare than the consequences of not having an airway when one is needed.

So I tubed him.

By now there were three nurses assisting me. While the other two continued to prevent my patient from hurting himself, I asked the third to open the kit containing the equipment needed for intubation so I could make sure that the necessary equipment was present and working. (That was for my benefit, as the staff tested it independently every day.) I asked the respiratory therapist to put high-flow oxygen on him and leave it on until I was ready to pass the tube; I elected not to give him extra medication as I didn't think any others would be of use; and I had already done a rapid assessment for potential difficulties with the intubation, including the relationships with tongue, jaw, and chin. So I checked the light in the laryngoscope one more time, and then asked the nurse to push a 20 mg IV of etomidate, followed in a few seconds by a 100 mg IV of succinylcholine, and to start the clock. It is maybe worth noting that these two chemicals are similar to those used to execute people by lethal injection. This is not a procedure that is done casually. (The third medication used in lethal injection, potassium chloride, stops the heart as well. This particular feature is not considered to be desirable in rapid sequence intubation.)

Within thirty seconds, the etomidate was working: the

patient had relaxed completely and was on his way to a state of profound sedation in which he would not be aware of anything that was happening to him. During this time, we gently laid him flat on his back and put a small towel behind his head to move it slightly forward. While we did this, his eyes had a moment of twitching, which signaled that the paralytic was taking effect.

At approximately one minute following the succinylcholine, I judged him to be fully paralyzed. Tipping his head backward, I put the curved blade of the laryngoscope into his mouth and slid it past his tongue and into the vallecula, the space between the open trapdoor of the epiglottis and the back of the tongue. Then I lifted up on the handle of the laryngoscope. Usually when I do that, the epiglottis will also lift out of the way, allowing me to see the cords.

Not this time. In his case the epiglottis was just long and floppy enough that it just fell downward in front of the tracheal opening.

I asked about his oxygen saturation. "Still ninety-eight percent," said the respiratory therapist.

So I removed the laryngoscope with the curved blade and took the one with the long straight blade. This time instead of trying to insert the tip behind the epiglottis, I deliberately slid it past the epiglottis and the trachea into the esophagus—which is a very easy target. Next, I put my right hand on the patient's Adam's apple and gently pressed downward. Then, while holding upward pressure on the laryngoscope handle, I slowly slid the blade out again. Sure enough, just as it passed the tracheal opening, with its firm ring of cartilage, it dropped downward into my view. The epiglottis meanwhile now remained firmly trapped above it by the tip of the blade. At this point, as if they were the face of my wife on our wedding day, I kept my gaze fixed on those beautiful vocal cords. You can have your sunsets over the Grand Canyon, or your beautiful ocean views. I think many emergency physicians will agree with me when I say that—at least while doing a difficult intubation—there are few sights in the universe that match the beauty of a pair of vocal cords.

I asked the nurse to put his hand on the Adam's apple to maintain the pressure, and I reached my right hand backward to receive the endotracheal tube. It now had a long metal wire running down inside the barrel. It was flexible enough to be bent into any shape but firm enough to hold that shape during the procedure. It was used to make the tube curve just the right amount to go where it had to go. Slipping it into the right side of his mouth, I watched it curve upward and into the trachea. As soon as it was past the cords, I carefully pulled out the wire, asked the respiratory therapist to inflate the bulb, and then gave the tube over to his care, to fix in place, while I checked all the previously mentioned items and verified that indeed the tube was still where it was supposed to be.

His tube was fine. And when I came back for my next shift in a few days, I learned that he had done well. The ICU physician had been able to discharge him to a treatment program the next day. I was not surprised to learn that he had remembered nothing about his ER visit.

It's okay. I remembered for him.

CHAPTER FIFTEEN

Nova

HERE IS A picture: a young man sitting in a wheelchair, alert but confused. The back of his head is smeared with blood.

Just a couple of minutes before, he had walked into the ER and told the nurse at triage that he thought somebody had shot him. He had been in a nearby bar having a beer when he heard a loud noise and felt a hard blow to the back of his head. He had no idea why this had happened.

The nurse put him immediately into a wheelchair and rolled him back to the trauma room. I examined him where he sat. He was alert, with normal vital signs. From the front, it seemed as if nothing was wrong. But when I palpated the back of his skull, I found a small soft depression consistent with an entry wound. Just above it I felt an irregularity under the scalp.

I asked how he was feeling. He said that his head hurt but otherwise he didn't feel too bad. He could move his arms and legs normally and was talking without any difficulty, so the possibility that anything had actually penetrated his skull seemed unlikely. I guessed that perhaps, if he had been shot, it had been by a low-velocity weapon such as a pellet gun; that the projectile had struck the skull at an angle without enough energy to penetrate the bone; and instead it had tunneled up outside the bone but under the scalp, forming the lump that I could feel.

I told him what I suspected, but I needed to be sure, so I ordered a CT scan of his head. That way I could verify that my suspicion was correct, and also ensure that he had not injured his brain simply from the blunt trauma to his skull.

It was only fifteen or twenty minutes later when the tech took him back to the trauma room. The young man was now out of his wheelchair and lying on a gurney. He was still awake and able to answer questions. The tech had the films with him also. However, instead of just putting them on the desktop in front of the view screen, he handed them to me personally and then stood waiting, saying nothing. I took the films, snapped them into place on the view box, and took a look.

For a moment, I didn't understand what I was seeing. His brain looked completely normal. There was no sign of bleeding or swelling or any other kind of damage in either hemisphere. The lower portions of the brain were also intact. Even so, there was clearly something terribly wrong. Exactly in the middle of the brain—between the two uninjured hemispheres, and just above the intact midbrain—was a shining star.

In any other circumstance, it would have been beautiful. It had no obvious shape or form. It was simply a spot of utter whiteness surrounded by rays of light spreading outward in all directions into the surrounding brain.

I knew what it was, of course. It was the bullet. It had

struck him precisely in the center of the back of his skull, had gone into his brain . . . and stopped. It had somehow found its way into the very middle of the most complex object in the known universe—the human brain—without doing any observable damage.

It was probably a .22; that caliber has the right amount of power to penetrate the skull and still not obliterate the surrounding brain. It didn't look like a bullet, though. The radiation utilized by CT scanners passes through human tissue, but it will bounce off irregularly shaped metal objects. When it does so, it can produce artifacts on the film that look just like rays of light, like a star—a tiny nova—exploding in the middle of the brain.

I asked the nurse to page the neurosurgeon. He was in the hospital, and I told him what I thought was going on. Within a few minutes, he was standing beside me, looking at the CT scan. He agreed that except for the bullet in the center, the brain looked perfectly normal. The bullet had not "tunneled up the scalp"; instead it had entered the skull precisely between the two halves of his brain, just above the place where those two halves joined together to form the midbrain and spinal cord—and therefore in a place where there was really no brain tissue at all.

I turned to the neurosurgeon and asked what he could do. "Nothing," he said.

"Nothing?" I replied. "Doesn't he need to have it removed? He seems pretty neurologically intact."

"That's because the swelling hasn't gotten going. But it's too deep. He's going to die, and there is nothing I can do."

It had been an extraordinarily lucky—and unlucky—shot. The bullet itself had missed both the cerebral hemispheres and the midbrain. For a moment, he seemed fine. But the momentum of a bullet is not the same as a pair of gardener's shears. The inflammatory reaction and swelling from the bullet's impact were already causing the area around it to swell, cutting off the circulation to the midbrain, below the two hemispheres.

As he left the ER to go up to the neurosurgical ICU, he was already becoming confused. He died four hours later.

CHAPTER SIXTEEN

Last Rights

I T WAS LATE one winter afternoon. Or it would have been, if there really were such a thing as a winter afternoon in Georgia. I was called to the cardiac care room to see an elderly gentleman with a chief complaint of chest pain.

In medical terminology, the term "chief complaint" has a very precise meaning. Specifically, the chief complaint is what the patient answers when you ask why they came to the ER.

Some chief complaints attract more of a response than others. "I can't seem to shake this cold" generally yields some quiet time watching TV in the waiting room, while "I have been having chest pain" almost always results in a quick and intense response—especially if, as you say those words, you are holding a clenched fist over the middle of your chest.

That response is not because people with chest pain are necessarily having a heart attack; most are not. Rather, it's because people who are having a heart attack often complain of chest pain. Given that we see lots and lots of people, if we don't evaluate every such complaint rapidly, sooner or later someone will die while waiting to be seen.

We would have seen this patient quickly in any case; he

came by ambulance. (Not all people who come by ambulance are seriously ill. But enough of them are to justify an immediate triage evaluation—and generally a trip to the head of the line.) He had arrived with two small tubes in his nostrils, giving him extra oxygen. Immediately, he had been placed in one of the critical patient rooms, with three nurses caring for him. Now one of the nurses was starting an IV in his left arm and drawing blood samples, a second had opened his shirt and was attaching EKG leads to his chest and extremities, and a third was offering him a small paper cup containing baby aspirin, and asking him to chew them and then swallow. At that point, he had been in the ER maybe two minutes.

When I arrived, he did not appear to be in any discomfort. The ambulance note said he was an elderly gentleman, mildly overweight, describing himself as a nonsmoker, who had given his age as seventy-nine. All that appeared reasonable to me.

I did not have to ask him what he did for a living. He was dressed in a black shirt, pants, shoes, and socks. Around his neck, he wore a simple white collar and a gold chain from which a small crucifix was suspended.

I went over to the bed, took his right hand in mine, and shook it. As I did so, I said, "Hi. I'm Paul Seward. I'm one of the doctors here. How can I help you?"

He smiled calmly back at me. Then he said, "Hi. I'm Father Allen. I don't know, really. I was getting ready to go to dinner when I started getting a pain in my chest."

His demeanor was a little surprising. Most people who have been snatched from their ordinary lives and taken in an ambulance to an emergency room, and who, the moment they arrive, have all sorts of things pasted on them, stuck into them, shoved up their noses, and dumped in their mouths, are at least moderately concerned about what is going on. But Father Allen might as well have been watching an interesting TV show. I was probably more worried than he seemed to be.

However, just as it had for the nurses, the words "chest pain" opened a little imaginary file drawer in my mind, so I reached in and pulled out an invisible list of questions: What time did this pain begin? Did it come and go, or was it steady? Where exactly in your chest did you feel it? Did it extend somewhere else? Was it sharp? Achy? Burning? How bad was the pain when it started? Were you short of breath with the pain? Did you break a sweat? Is it still there? Is it worse now than it was? Or the same? Or improving? And so forth.

With each question and each answer, a picture emerged.

He was indeed a retired Episcopal priest. For many years, he had worked in this community as the pastor of a local church. However, he also had a degree in social work, and throughout that time, he had also been closely involved with a local community mental health center, working one day a week as a volunteer counselor. His wife had died about ten years ago, so five years later when he retired, he had moved to the Midwest to be closer to his only other relative, an older brother. But then, a year ago, his brother had died, and now he lived alone.

But something exciting had happened: the mental health center where he had worked had decided to have a reception and a dinner, to celebrate the fiftieth anniversary of its opening. Former employees from all over the country were coming back for the event, some to be recognized for their years of service. Father Allen was one of them. Equally important, several of the people who worked at the center were former parishioners, so he was certain that at the dinner he would see many friends whom he had not seen in years.

And then, this.

He had been at his hotel getting dressed for the event when the pain started. At first it was minor, like a little indigestion. However, over a few minutes it became worse. At the same time, he found himself starting to be a little short of breath and had to sit down. He described the pain not as sharp but as more of an ache or a pressure, a little like something was tight in his chest. As he said these words, he put his hand over his breastbone, made a fist, and squeezed—just a little.

At that point, he had realized that this might be something worse than indigestion, so he called some friends who had also returned for the celebration and were also staying at the hotel. He asked if they could come to his room to help him.

His friends were there in minutes. By that time, though the pain was about the same, it had extended upward toward his left jaw—almost like a toothache. They immediately called 911.

The ambulance arrived quickly. The EMTs assessed him, put him on some oxygen, and placed him in the ambulance. The oxygen seemed to help his breathing, and at the same time the pain eased somewhat. They also gave him a small tablet of nitroglycerin under his tongue. It burned a little but the paramedic said that was okay, it just meant that it was working. (When placed under the tongue, nitroglycerin is absorbed rapidly into the bloodstream, where it opens the blood vessels and allows the heart to have an easier time doing its job. The burning is from the dilation of the blood vessels in the tongue.) Father Allen thought that was interesting.

However, he said, it never did get unbearable. When the EMTs asked him to rate it on a scale of one to ten, he had given it a five. En route he continued to feel better, and by the time he got to the hospital the pain was gone. Now he said that he felt perfectly normal.

Then he asked, "Do you think I can go back to the hotel now? I don't want to be late for dinner."

I think I might have grimaced a little, but I confess I was not very surprised. When someone's life is unexpectedly invaded by a serious illness, denial is a standard response. Therefore, if the illness might be a heart attack, we will ask the doctor if that means we won't be able to play golf next Sunday. That's not because we don't know what a heart attack is. It's just an indirect way of asking if we have heard the doctor correctly. It can't be that serious, can it?

This was all the more true for Father Allen. He had just traveled over a thousand miles to visit with, and be recognized by, friends he had not seen in years. The value of a lifetime of work was going to be acknowledged. How could he be lying in a hospital bed a few miles away while that was happening? He didn't want to be having a heart attack. He wanted it to be indigestion. Or a toothache. Something that might do just fine with a little Alka-Seltzer.

But I couldn't say that.

Instead I said, "I'm sorry." I went on: "The problem is that you have a very good history for someone who could be having a serious heart problem, and we need to do a few tests so we can be sure of what's going on."

He nodded thoughtfully as he—perhaps unconsciously—touched his crucifix with his hand. Then he looked at me. "How long do you think that will take?"

"Not too long," I replied. "I need to take a good look at your electrocardiogram first. Also, the blood work should be back in twenty or thirty minutes."

He looked briefly at his watch. Then he smiled. "Okay. I can wait. Can my friends come in now?"

"Of course," I said.

In a couple of minutes, three men dressed in business suits entered the room and came over to him. One of them put a hand on his arm. Another turned to me.

"May we ask how things are?" he said.

I looked at Father Allen. He nodded and then added, "Of course you can. You can tell them anything. These are my friends."

So I told them what I thought was happening. I said that his history was strongly suggestive of either a heart attack or at the very least a new onset of angina. The tests I was doing—the cardiogram and the blood tests—were to see whether I could distinguish which one was happening, though both were quite serious events.

They nodded. I don't expect patients to understand everything I say the first time around, but I figured that when the test results came back, that would be an opportunity to go over everything again—this time with a better idea of what was going on.

At that point, the nurse handed me the EKG. It was normal. Given his history, I was not surprised; people will generally have no EKG findings after a new angina attack. Perhaps the blood vessel had opened again just by itself. Perhaps the nitro had eased the work of the heart enough that the flow was sufficient. Perhaps it had been just a temporary spasm. Lots of possibilities.

Then, a few minutes later, the blood tests came back. They were normal too. Again, that was not a surprise.

I felt good about the results. Here was a healthy older man who, almost certainly, had just had his first attack of angina. On the one hand, that meant that he had a dangerously unstable condition that could worsen at any time; but on the other hand, he had gotten safely here to the hospital, alive and well, with an undamaged heart. All that was left to do was to give him some medicine to control his heart rate and to keep him from making more clots in his coronaries, and admit him to an observation bed. Then the cardiologist could come in tomorrow morning and decide what to do next.

So I put together the lab slips and the EKG and went back to his room. He was still comfortably waiting on the gurney, IVs in place, EKG leads still stuck on his chest, monitor still running, and talking about old times at the rehab center with his friends.

He looked up and smiled. "What's the report? Am I having a heart attack?"

"Well, not exactly," I said. Then I pulled over a chair and sat down next to him. "May I talk in front of your friends?" I asked.

Once more he smiled and said, "Of course."

So I did. I went over the history of his pain and why I was concerned. I talked about angina and how it wasn't a heart attack, but it often meant that a real heart attack was just around the corner; that in fact, untreated, the death rate within one week is about the same from new-onset, unstable angina as it is from a true heart attack.

He nodded in agreement, and then said, "So that means I need to come back tomorrow to see the heart specialist?"

"Uh, no," I said. "It means that I need to admit you to a special part of the hospital where we can watch you overnight, monitor your heart, and make sure that if your pain comes back, it doesn't progress to something more serious."

He now had a more thoughtful expression. "I see," he said. "What do you mean by 'more serious'?"

"Well, there are several possibilities. First, if the blood supply in one of the arteries in your heart shuts down, it can damage or kill the heart muscle that it supplies. That can weaken your heart and cause heart failure."

He nodded again, still seeming more like someone taking a class in school than someone talking about his own heart. "Is that the worst?"

I was dancing around the d-word. Doctors often do. We don't like the d-word. It is our enemy, one we fight against every day. And sooner or later we always lose. But it was time to use it.

"Well, no," I said, "you could die."

I paused just for a second, just to be sure he had heard me. Then I continued.

"If the heart muscle and the nerves in the heart become seriously injured, then the nerves in the heart can fire in the wrong places or at the wrong times. That can cause a condition called ventricular fibrillation. In that situation, the heart doesn't beat at all; it just wiggles a little. When that happens, if no one is nearby with the equipment and training to correct it, you will become unconscious in a matter of seconds, and in a few minutes, you will be dead."

There, I thought. *I said it twice. Did he get it now?*

He did.

"Ah," he said, and then nodded as if he were thinking things over. Then he looked back at me, still with the expression of a student discussing a problem in cardiovascular physiology.

"So either nothing happens and I come back after dinner. Or I start having pain again and I come back immediately. Or I might just die? Is that right?"

"Pretty much—except for the fourth possibility, which is staying here. Then you will almost certainly be fine."

He nodded again. But then he said, "But then I miss dinner." Now he was the one talking to me as if I didn't understand something obvious.

I was surprised. This was not a patient in denial. This was a patient who had completely accepted what was happening to him—and was still not sure he wanted treatment. That was not an answer I had ever gotten in such a serious situation. "That's . . . true," I said. "But . . . is a dinner as important as your life?"

He smiled. "Look at it my way," he said. "I'm an old man. I have some cholesterol problems, and I take medicine for high blood pressure. I suspect that no matter what I do, I will be back here, or somewhere like this, in the not-very-distant future."

He stopped for a moment. Then his expression changed. He was no longer relaxed and smiling but thoughtful and earnest. "Let me try to explain. I worked for most of my life at the rehab center and at the church. These"—he gestured at the other three men—"are my closest lifelong friends. I live alone now. But tonight, we are going to a dinner with people who we have known for a very long time, where we are all going to celebrate one another and being together." Then he shook his head slightly. "And that will never happen again."

I looked up at his friends. They stood around him quietly, not smiling. Nor did they say anything in disagreement.

So I looked back at Father Allen. "Then do you want to leave the hospital?" I said it as a question, but I already knew the answer.

"It's not that I don't want to stay in the hospital," he said. "It's that I do want to go to dinner."

I sat still for a minute. Then I asked the three men, "Does he really mean this? Do you understand the risk he is taking?" They looked at him. Then one of them nodded. "Yes, I am sure he does," he said.

"Okay," I said, "I am going to go do a brief errand. Will you all talk about all this, and make sure that you all understand—and especially that you understand, Father Allen—the risk you are asking to take? Then I will come back, and we will have another talk."

I gave them about ten minutes. When I came back, I had a form in my hand entitled "Leaving Against Medical Advice." It's the form we use when people choose to refuse care. It's not that uncommon a choice. But almost always, when patients do choose to leave against advice, it's either because of a less serious medical problem or because they don't really believe what we are saying.

But Father Allen knew exactly what I was saying. He understood that it was true. That was a new one for me.

The form already had a lot of printed words on it—but I had added several lines specifically detailing how dangerous a decision this was. I also had indicated a place for his friends to sign, attesting that they thought he was in his right mind and understood what he was doing. I went over it in detail. Then Father Allen signed it, as did each of his friends.

As I did so, I noted that while I was out of the room, he had redressed himself in his clerical attire.

When they had all finished signing, I shook his hand and said, "Please don't wait till something happens. Come back as soon as you can." He smiled and said he would.

I didn't know what else to say. I just said, "I hope you have a very nice evening."

Evidently, he did. I was off duty that night, but when I came back in the morning, the first thing I asked was whether he had returned to be readmitted.

The charge nurse on duty said that well, not exactly. According to his friends, who had called the hospital to let us know what had happened, he did indeed have a very good time talking to old friends, eating a good meal, and being thanked for what he had done with his life. Then he said that he was tired and wanted to go back to his hotel and get a good night's sleep. He promised that he would go to the hospital in the morning.

Over the years, I have often thought of the choice he made, to go back to the hotel instead of returning to the ER after dinner; what choice he was really making. Because the next day, he did not answer his friends' knock. The desk clerk had to let them in.

They found Father Allen in bed. He had evidently died peacefully a few hours before.

CHAPTER SEVENTEEN

Last Wrongs

I N THE EMERGENCY department, most patients are new
to us. We pick up a chart from the rack and review the
vital signs and chief complaint. If it looks as if it might be
a complicated problem, we check quickly for an old chart,
either for a brief once-over or simply to be sure it is there.
Then we head to whichever room or gurney they occupy, to
meet them for the first time. I have written a little about the
things I try to do to help patients feel safe, comfortable, and
perhaps more trusting of what is happening to them.

That being said, on this particular day, this very particular patient could not have cared less whether I shook her
hand, played the fiddle, or danced a jig. She had her own
long-standing opinion about what our professional relationship would be, and as far as she was concerned, that opinion
ruled.

For starters, she had no doubt about who understood her
problem the best: she did. Similarly, she knew precisely what
would constitute a correct and acceptable treatment for that
problem. In her mind, my job was only to implement the decisions she had already made and to do so with as little bother
as possible.

She was not entirely irrational in this belief. Although she lived in a skilled nursing facility and was in her mideighties, she was a retired nurse—one who had spent most of her career in that very hospital, in senior positions that included one in the emergency department. She didn't tell me outright that when she started working there, I had been too young to spell "emergency," but I sensed that the thought was in her mind.

When I greeted her, her response was polite but terse. And when I began to ask her about her medical history, she asked in return whether I had read her chart, and if I hadn't, then what was I doing standing there talking to her?

I nodded at this, and said that I usually liked to get a sense of what was going on first, so that when I looked at the old chart, I would have a better idea of what I was looking for.

She humphed at that and then said that she would keep it simple, her expression implying that she would do so to ensure that a simpleton like myself could understand it. She told me that her underlying problem was congestive heart failure; that she was managed on a couple of diuretics (which help draw off the excess fluid that the heart is having trouble pumping around) plus digoxin (an old medicine that helps the heart beat more strongly); and that normally she did well, but for the last few days she had begun to have some increased shortness of breath while walking, and a bit more so when lying flat. These are signs that the heart is not beating strongly enough to take the fluid out of the lungs. Usually when that happened, her doctor (a local, very reputable internist) would give her a shot of Lasix (a strong diuretic that is very good at getting rid of extra water but can take away important electrically active minerals—particularly sodium and potassium—that are involved in maintaining the rhythm of the heart), and that would take care of it. However, he was out of town and she didn't like the doctor who was taking his calls (I was able to conceal my astonishment at this revelation), so she came here to get it—and that was what she wanted.

I nodded and said that all that seemed to make sense. However, as this was the first time I had seen her, I had to make sure for myself, and would she mind if I examined her? She shrugged and said nothing, which I took for acquiescence. She let me listen to her lungs and heart, check pulses, and look for swelling in her lower extremities. She even let me examine her abdomen to see whether there was any sign of liver enlargement. Finally, I asked if she minded if I got a little blood for some lab work as well as a chest X-ray and cardiogram.

"Why?" she asked. "You listened to my lungs, my pulse ox is normal, and you know what I have." By "pulse ox," she meant a measurement of blood oxygen level, taken from a clip on the finger that calculates the oxygen level from the color of the blood.

I decided that my best chance was to respect her knowledge and address it rather than challenge it. So I did something I try never to do: I answered in doctor talk and assumed that she spoke it fluently.

"You are on daily hydrochlorothiazide, a diuretic that

wastes potassium. So does Lasix. You also take digoxin. That means I need at least to know your potassium and digoxin levels to be sure you are not setting yourself up for a dangerous arrhythmia." Elevated levels of digoxin make heart arrhythmia due to potassium problems even more likely. She thought for a moment. Then she said, "Okay. You can get the X-ray and the electrolytes and the EKG. Then I want some Lasix. And then I want to go home. You know that you don't need the dig level if my potassium is normal and my EKG is okay."

She was correct. She was in her eighties, living in a nursing home, and was giving me lessons in cardiology, pharmacology, and physiology.

"Okay, it's a deal," I said, and wrote the orders. Twenty minutes later I had looked at an EKG that showed no signs of toxic levels of digoxin and no changes from her previous tracings, and a chest X-ray that indicated mild heart failure and normal electrolytes. I gave her the Lasix and sent her home.

And that was that. I had actually enjoyed her visit, in a masochistic sort of way. It is refreshing to see patients who take complete responsibility for their own care. But I never expected any follow-up.

However, about two or three months later, a little after noon, we got a radio call that the EMTs were a block away and en route with an elderly woman with no pulse and an unknown down time. She was unresponsive and not breathing on her own, her heart rhythm was ventricular fibrillation, and CPR was in progress. They had attempted defibrillation once and were trying to start an IV.

By now you know that such a call is not uncommon. You also know that most of the time, when patients come in who are not breathing and have no heartbeat, it is because they are dead.

Even so, we always try to give them the benefit of the doubt. So when we got her into the resuscitation room, we continued CPR, gave her some IV epinephrine and some amiodarone (a drug that suppresses abnormal heart rhythms), and shocked her some more. During this process, I also intubated her, to protect our ability to breathe for her.

To my surprise, it worked. Suddenly, after the second or third shock, she converted to a normal rhythm on the monitor, with a strong pulse at the wrist to go with it. She had a decent blood pressure. And her color was improving. It appeared as if we might indeed have dragged her body back from the dead. It was time to examine her more closely to see whether we had brought a functional person back with it.

It was not a happy examination. Her eyes did not respond to light, and she did not respond in any way to shouted words, or to pinching her shoulder muscle or rubbing on her chest bone with my knuckles. In short, she scored no higher on tests for a functioning brain than would a department store mannequin or a statue in the park.

Yet despite all that, for the moment she was stable. The respiratory therapist had put her on a ventilator, which was breathing for her; her vital signs were good; and her heart was beating steadily and well. There was nothing more we could do for her in the emergency room. It was time to send her upstairs to the intensive care unit to see if they had anything that they could offer. So for the first time since her arrival, I sat down at the physician's work station, reached for the old chart, and began to read. The moment I did so, I recognized her name and remembered our prior encounter.

Unfortunately, that was not all I realized.

Did I mention above that in general, emergency physicians do not see their patients more than once? I should have known that she would be an exception. And I might have predicted that once more I would fail her by not having read her chart.

Just below her name, on the very first page, in handwriting that was as firm and clear as she herself had been when she was alive, was the instruction that should she present to the hospital in cardiac arrest, under *no circumstances* was she to be resuscitated. Specifically, that meant no CPR, no defibrillation, and no assisting of her ventilations. In addition, she absolutely refused to allow anyone to put a tube into her windpipe and breathe for her, if otherwise she could not.

As I read, I could see her in my mind's eye, shaking her head at the sad fact that in the hour of her greatest need, she had gotten me for her doctor. Because, of course, I had just done every one of the things that she had not wanted to be done. Worse yet, because I had done all of them, the fears that had led her to this declaration had come true: her body was alive, with a good heartbeat and blood pressure, but her brain was almost certainly dead. And even if by some incredible chance, there was still some life inside, I had still disobeyed every instruction she had given. What to do now?

There was only one thing I could do: I could obey her last remaining instruction. I looked at the end of the document for the name of her health care proxy, what in the old days we used to call "next of kin."

It turned out to be her son. He lived not far from the hospital. The chart even listed his phone number at work. So I asked the nursing staff to move her to a side room with some privacy, and while they were doing so, I called him. I told him that his mother had come in with a cardiac arrest and was near death. He was calm and unsurprised. I think it was a call he had been expecting. Then I told him what had happened—that she had come in in full arrest, that I had not had—or at least had not taken—the time to check her chart. I went on to say that because I had not known her wishes, we had resuscitated her but had succeeded only in bringing her heart back but not her brain. Only after reading her chart did I realize that she had strongly wanted to avoid the condition she was now in. I asked if he wanted to come to the emergency department, both to see her and to help us decide what to do next. He said he would be there in about forty-five minutes.

Long before he arrived, I decided what I would suggest.

It seemed to me that we had only one option left that would let us follow as closely as possible the intent of the instructions in her living will. In those instructions, her clearest wish was that she did not want to be helped to breathe; if she needed that, then she would rather be dead.

So when her son arrived, I suggested that we honor that

request. I would take her off the ventilator and attach the ET tube instead to a "T piece." This was a T-shaped tube designed so that oxygen from the hospital wall supply could flow either into her endotracheal tube or out into the room. There was nothing that would prevent her from breathing—if she could. Her airway was open and protected, and there was plenty of oxygen to breathe. But if she did not breathe on her own, there would no longer be anything to force her to do so. Furthermore, if he wanted to, he could sit with her for as long as he wished, as we waited for the outcome.

I was also very clear with him that I thought that it extremely unlikely that she would take any breaths on her own, as she had made no attempt to do so since she was first seen by the EMTs from the ambulance. I also said that if this was the case, in a few minutes, her heart, deprived of oxygen, would slow down and either go into ventricular fibrillation or simply cease to beat. He said that this choice was what she would have wanted.

We had left the patient attached to a cardiac monitor and a pulse oximeter to measure the amount of oxygen in her bloodstream. At the moment, it registered nearly 100 percent—all her blood cells had as much oxygen as they could hold. I had arranged the curtain so that I could see the numbers and the tracing on the screen, but her son would not have to do so. That was okay with him. It only took a few seconds to detach the ventilator and replace it with the T piece. Then her son sat down in a chair by the head of the bed and held her hand. I told him that I would be nearby, then stepped out and pulled the curtain. The wait was not short. I remember checking the screen frequently, watching the percentage of oxygen in her blood drop lower and lower, while the sharply pointed electrical waves marking her heartbeat marched across the screen with the strict regularity of a drill team.

Five minutes; then ten. Below 90 percent the oxygen level starts to drop more rapidly. At 80 percent, most people who are not acclimatized to high altitudes will not survive for long.

But no one seemed to have informed her heart of this. I imagined the disciplined muscle fibers that together comprised her heart, snorting with laughter at the thought that a little oxygen deprivation might keep them from doing their job.

When the clock reached fifteen minutes and the oxygen saturation was down in the low fifties, I sat for a few minutes with her son as he held his mother's hand. As I did so, I felt her pulse. It was faint and thready, but I could still count it. I explained to him that this was taking longer than I had expected and asked how he was doing. He said he was okay with it. He had known his mother well, and the fact that her heart was giving death a run for its money was not a surprise. Between fifteen and twenty minutes, when the oxygen saturation was in the low forties and rapidly approaching the thirties, her heart started to falter. As her heartbeat slowed, the spikes of electricity, visible on her monitor, ceased being sharp mountain peaks and gradually became soft, rounded hills. At that point, I quietly checked for her pulse again. She no longer had one. I told her son that it was over. Gently, he placed her hand on her chest. Then, as he had left instructions for the release of her body to the funeral director and had no more questions, he said thank you and left.

I turned off the monitor, disconnected the leads, and went back to work.

CHAPTER EIGHTEEN

Graduation

UNIVERSITY HOSPITAL HAD lots of roles. One of them was to be the nighttime morgue. If someone died unexpectedly, outside the hospital, the bodies were taken to the county medical examiner's office. But at night, when the county offices were closed, they came to us.

The ER had a little room that had been a storage closet, just outside the main patient care area. It was there that, at night, the EMTs took the bodies of people they could not save. Then the nighttime charge nurse would make a call to the coroner, Leroy Sims, and somewhere between a few minutes and an hour or so later, he would wander in, perhaps get a cup of coffee, stop and say hello to the people who were working that night, and then go look at the bodies.

He was an older man, a bit overweight, with a rumbling bass voice that would befit an opera singer. He was a good man—in my book, another unnoticed hero. He had been a coroner for many years, and before that a homicide detective. Thus he had spent his life looking daily at terrible things, making difficult decisions, and delivering the worst of news to devastated strangers, in as kind a manner as he could. He was also a gifted organist, who would often go home after work and play the organ to ease the pain of what he had coped with that day.

He did his job well. Others also thought him a good man. After his death, the Georgia Coroners Association created an award for service that bears his name.

On this night, sometime in early May, the body in the back room was that of a teenaged boy, a senior at a local high school. He and a friend had been driving home from an evening activity related to the end of the school year. The vehicle had rolled over several times. The driver had had his seat belt on and was evidently uninjured. At least he had not come to our care.

The passenger—this young man—had not been belted. Furthermore—it was a warm spring evening—the window on his side was open, and when the rollover occurred, he was ejected through the side window onto the ground and crushed by the rolling car. According to the EMTs, he was dead when they arrived.

Sometime later, Mr. Sims arrived. I don't remember why I joined him, but I remember standing together in the tiny nighttime morgue on opposite sides of the gurney. One of us had unzipped the bag. Because the boy was still fully dressed, his major injuries—crushing damage to the chest, abdomen, pelvis—were not visible, and if you looked with eyes half-closed, he did not look terribly different than perhaps he had looked a few hours earlier when he was still alive: a young man with a tie, a dress shirt, and a blue blazer. Only now he was lying on a gurney with his eyes closed.

He had a couple of pieces of paper sticking out of his breast pocket.

I reached over and took them out, examining them for a moment. Then I showed them to the coroner. "Graduation tickets," he said, and shook his head. He zipped up the bag, and we left the room.

Even though it was late, I am sure he had a cup of coffee before he left. Then, I have no doubt, he went home to play the organ for a while before he went to sleep.

CHAPTER NINETEEN

An Ordinary Day

A BLACK CAT should have run across the road while I was driving to work that day. Instead, it was on an ordinary day, in the middle of an ordinary shift, when a man, who had awoken that morning feeling reasonably well, became my patient and then, despite everything I knew how to do, went on to die. I am sure that he had not expected to die that day. And when I greeted him, neither did I. But then, most people die on ordinary days when they are not expecting to do so.

He had come to the ER because of increasing shortness of breath. This was no surprise as he frequently came to the ER for help with this problem. He had two serious lung diseases, asthma and COPD, and even at his best he was a little short of breath.

Asthma, or reactive airway disease as it is more precisely called, is a problem in which the muscles that surround the bronchioles (the smallest air passages in the lungs) are unusually sensitive to allergens and irritants. They react by squeezing down too much, making the bronchioles too narrow. When this happens, inhaling is not affected very much, because the overall expansion of our chests and lungs makes these passages larger. But when an asthmatic tries to exhale, these passages are compressed even further, making the outward flow of air more difficult. This narrowing causes the patient's exhalation to be accompanied by a soft, high-pitched hissing noise, which we call wheezing.

COPD, or chronic obstructive pulmonary disease, is a single term for two lung problems that commonly occur together. The first is chronic bronchitis, which refers to a long-term inflammation of the bronchioles in the lungs. The second is emphysema, which is a similar inflammation and destruction of the alveoli. Alveoli are the small sacs of air at the ends of the bronchioles where the bloodstream and the air are separated by only a thin membrane, allowing oxygen (the fuel for our metabolism) to diffuse into the bloodstream, and carbon dioxide (the waste product of our metabolism) to diffuse out.

In short, he had two diseases—asthma and chronic bronchitis—that interfered with the passage of air in and out of his lungs, and a third, emphysema, that was damaging the places where the air needed to go.

However, other than that, he was about as healthy as a middle-aged, two-pack-a-day smoker can expect to be.

I recall him as being in his midfifties, though looking about ten years older than he was, moderately graying of hair and wrinkled of skin. Like many people with COPD, he was somewhat barrel-chested. (The inability to breathe out well means that their lungs are permanently more full of air than they should be, causing their chest to be more rounded, like a barrel.) He appeared to be moderately short of breath, but no worse than on other occasions when I had cared for him.

Even so, because of his breathing problems, the triage nurse had put him in one of the rooms designed for critical patients, and asked me to come see him as soon as possible. When I entered the room, he was still fully dressed, sitting on a chair and removing his shoes. In his front shirt pocket were the two telltale signs of his diseases: a pack of cigarettes and a medication inhaler.

I gave him a hand, helping him with his shirt and tying his gown in back, and in a minute or so he was seated on the gurney. The part that supported his back was tipped upward as far as it would go, allowing him to rest but at the same time still sit upright. People who are having difficulty breathing for almost any reason nearly always need to sit up. Lying down makes the contents of their abdomen press upon their diaphragm, which makes breathing more difficult. Also, if there is any fluid in their lungs, sitting up helps it to settle to the bottom. The nurse had done one set of vital signs and began putting in an IV. He had also clipped a pulse oximeter onto the tip of one of the patient's fingers.

All things considered, his vitals were not terribly out of line. His heart rate was up a bit, around 110, and his blood pressure was in the high normal range. Neither of these was surprising considering the extra effort that it cost him to breathe and the fact that he had already taken several puffs from his albuterol inhaler. Albuterol is a common trade name for salbutamol, a commonly used beta-agonist. These medications are used in patients with COPD and/or asthma to relax the muscles that shrink the bronchioles, making it easier for such patients to breathe. A common side effect is making the heart beat faster. Years ago, shots of adrenaline, also called epinephrine, were routinely used for the same effect.

His respiratory rate was around sixteen breaths per minute, which was within normal limits for his age. However, the way he was breathing was not normal. It was a combination of brief, rapid inhalations, followed by longer, slower exhalations.

Of greatest concern was the fact that his pO_2—that is, his blood oxygen saturation—was only around 91 percent. I knew that because of his disease, he lived all the time with a lower blood oxygen level than normal and was used to it. Even so, that fact gave him little reserve to fall back on when things got worse.

At that point, I asked the nurse to put him on oxygen and include an albuterol nebulization treatment. He did so, using a dilute mixture of albuterol, which he put in a small chamber attached to an oxygen mask. This system increased the oxygen he was breathing from the normal 20 percent found in room air to around 50 percent, and at the same time allowed the medicine to be taken up continually, as a breathable mist.

I took a brief history—lifelong smoker, two packs a day; asthma as a child, which went away in early adulthood but had recurred ten or fifteen years ago. Since that time, besides the asthma, he had developed some gradually worsening COPD. He had no other medical problems and was on no other medications.

I listened to his lungs and heart, noting reasonably good air movement despite the wheeze, and normal heart sounds. I wrote orders for some basic blood tests, a chest X-ray to be done with a portable machine so he would not have to leave the examination room, and an electrocardiogram. Finally, I asked for him to be given a strong anti-inflammatory medication in the steroid family, 40 mg of methylprednisolone via his IV. Also, mostly because of the pO_2, I asked the nurse to stay with the patient and to call me when the labs and X-ray were back. Then I went on to see someone else.

At least I think I did. I don't really remember. I didn't go to lunch; I wouldn't have left the ER when I had a patient with a significant breathing problem that I had just started to evaluate. But I could have easily taken care of a minor problem in a nearby room. I don't even remember whether the nurse called me back to see him again or I just went back on my own after giving the medications a little while to work.

I do remember that when I did check on him a short time later, he was worse. His pO_2 was holding at 90-91, but his respiratory rate was creeping up and he was plainly working harder to breathe. Now when he spoke, he did so in broken sentences—a few words, followed by a hard breath and then a few more. And he was already on the maximum oxygen I could give him by face mask alone.

This surprised me. While COPD and asthma are serious problems, they generally respond at least partially to acute treatment. A dose of steroids, a couple of albuterol treatments, a period of observation, and usually patients are breathing better. It is unusual to see these problems become worse in front of me.

For the first time, I began to seriously worry about him. I checked his labs: Normal blood count except for a moderate elevation in the number of the oxygen-carrying red cells in his blood. (The body does this commonly in people who chronically deliver less oxygen to the blood: if the trucks aren't full, then make more trucks.) The EKG was also normal except for the moderately rapid heartbeat. The enzyme tests that help look for a subtle heart attack as a precipitating cause were negative as well.

The chest X-ray was not normal: his chest was larger than usual, and his lungs were very translucent. Again, this was not a surprise. The alveoli are like millions of tiny balloons. They make up most of the volume of the lung, and so there is not much actual tissue to block the X-rays. However, his alveoli, as balloons, were as fully inflated as they could possibly be, making his lungs even more transparent than usual.

But I saw no sign of pneumonia or heart failure, or any sign of a collapse of a lung.

He was getting worse. For the moment, his oxygen was adequate. But I was becoming more worried about what might be happening to his carbon dioxide levels.

We breathe for two reasons: to bring in the groceries, and to take out the trash. First, we need to take in oxygen. But we also need to get rid of carbon dioxide, and people who have trouble breathing out will often have considerably more difficulty blowing out the carbon dioxide than sucking in the oxygen. In fact, many people with COPD, like my patient, have significantly elevated levels of carbon dioxide in their bloodstream all the time. The problem with this carbon dioxide excess is that it may lead them to breathe *less* than they really need to.

People are often surprised to learn that the signal to the brain that we need to take a breath is not low oxygen; it is high carbon dioxide. This is a good thing because it triggers the next breath while we still have ample oxygen; this way we don't go around all day with our oxygen level dropping every few seconds.

However, if we *always* have elevated carbon dioxide, then our brain becomes used to it, and it will not so readily trigger a breath. At this point, we may feel a need to breathe only when our oxygen gets low.

But the problem can be worse than just low oxygen levels. Some people with COPD may completely switch over to a system in which they are no longer sensitive to carbon dioxide levels at all, but only to low oxygen. The danger in this case is that if we give them extra oxygen, they may no longer feel the need to breathe frequently enough to get rid of their carbon dioxide, causing the carbon dioxide level of their blood to go up rapidly and dangerously.

What is wrong with too much carbon dioxide? The problem is that when it is dissolved in the blood, carbon dioxide turns into an acid, and acidosis—elevated acid levels in the blood—is poisonous. It impairs the ability of the cells in the body to carry out their chemical duties—including essential ones such as the normal beating of the heart. In the brain, this shows up as confusion, sedation, and a decreased urge to breathe, which leads to further carbon dioxide elevation, further acidosis, and so on—a vicious downward spiral in which death quickly becomes inevitable.

My patient was already on the maximum oxygen I could

give him by a face mask. So far he showed no signs of carbon dioxide poisoning. That is, he was alert and working hard to breathe. But even so, he was reaching a point at which his fatigue, the problems he must have had in sensing when to breathe, and the progression of his breathing difficulty meant that I could no longer trust him to breathe adequately on his own. It was time to decide whether I should intubate him and take over his breathing for him.

If it was at all possible to avoid it, I didn't want to intubate him. Even to attempt it would be dangerous. A patient near the edge of carbon dioxide acidosis cannot tolerate any interruption in his breathing—certainly not the minute or so it takes for the sedation and paralysis to work. Even if the intubation is successful, the patient may sustain so much additional lung damage from the pressures that are needed that he might never be able to breathe on his own again.

So I looked for some straws to grasp. One such straw was to give him an IV of two grams of magnesium. The evidence for this as a treatment for asthma or COPD was minimal, but I had already used the best options. I also gave him another large dose of steroids, trying for whatever anti-inflammatory effect I could get. I thought about giving him aminophylline. Early in my career, this used to be the standard medication for severe asthma. However, over the years, evidence had mounted that its benefits were outweighed by its side effects, particularly in COPD.

Nothing worked.

Now there was no way to avoid it. I paged the respiratory therapist and asked her to set up to intubate him. At the same time, I took a ventilation bag attached to an oxygen supply and a face mask that would seal tightly to his face. Next, I carefully explained to the patient what I was going to do, and asked him if he was okay with it. He was sweating now, not talking at all, and simply nodded quickly. Leaving him sitting, I lowered the entire gurney toward the floor a little so that I could stand behind him on a step stool and lean over the top of the gurney to reach his face. Then, taking off his basic oxygen mask, I held the ventilation mask in both hands and slowly and gently lowered it over his face. Once there, I held it securely, pressing his head back against the mattress for support. At the same time, the respiratory therapist began squeezing the bag in time with the patient's breathing.

For a while it seemed to work. Within a few seconds the patient began to relax a little and allowed the therapist to do the work for him. His oxygen saturation even crept up a little to 92 or 93 percent. And for about ten minutes that was what we did.

But it wasn't enough. We tried two or three times to wean him from the mask, but each time his distress returned in force, and it was clear that he was becoming very tired.

It was time for a tube. But how could I do it without killing him? At this point, even laying him flat might worsen his breathing enough to shut him down on the spot.

So I put it in his nose.

Nowadays, with better techniques and tools, nasotracheal intubation has gone out of fashion, but in those days, in similar situations, I found it a great help. It had several important advantages. First, it is something that one could do—indeed could only do—with a patient who was sitting up and breathing on his own. Second, it did not require paralysis or sedation. That meant that there would be no pause in his breathing while doing the procedure. And finally, if it took a little longer than expected, or even if I failed to get the tube in, I would not have made him worse.

By then his eyes were mostly closed as he worked to breathe. He opened them briefly as I explained what I needed to do, and then once more he nodded and closed his eyes. I don't know whether he understood me or even heard me.

The technique is simple to describe, if tricky to perform. First, I replaced his oxygen mask. However, instead of albuterol in his nebulizer, I put a couple of cc's of 2 percent lidocaine (a numbing agent). By now he was mostly mouth breathing, but I knew that some of it would come through his nose.

Next, I took some lubricating jelly that had been permeated with lidocaine, squeezed a glob of it directly up and into his right nostril, and rapidly rubbed the side of his nose to smear it around. By now, virtually all his breathing was through his mouth, and he barely seemed to notice. Then I took an endo-tracheal tube that was slightly smaller than I would normally use for an adult male and lubricated the outside of the barrel generously with more lidocaine jelly. Finally, still standing directly behind him, I slid the tube as gently as possible into his right nostril and allowed the curve in the tube to guide it backward and downward into the back of his throat, toward the tracheal opening. When I saw a little fog appear on the inside of the tube, I knew that some of the air from his lungs was going in and out through it. At that point, I knew that I was almost there.

Then I stopped.

I need to pause here. Some of you must be wondering how this kind of blind technique could possibly succeed. Didn't I spend an entire chapter discussing how utterly impossible it is to get past all the mechanisms we have for keeping solid objects out of our windpipe? And now I'm just going to shove it down his nose and expect it to go into the right place?

In fact, it usually works. It does so for two reasons. First, you might remember that most of those barriers to passing an ET tube through the mouth involve the tongue and muscles in the back of the throat. But by coming down from the nose, the tube has sneaked behind all those obstacles. Second, I told you about all the movements we must do to line the neck up in just the right position. However, when a person is having this much trouble breathing, he does the work for us. Instinctively, my patient had put his head forward, then tipped it upward and found the best position to make it as easy as possible for the air to get in and out. All I had to do was follow the path he had created.

And I had to time it correctly.

That was why I had stopped just before the tracheal opening. For several seconds, I simply stood there, reaching with my right hand around the back of his head to hold the end of the tube, keeping my right ear next to the opening. I listened carefully as he breathed rapidly in and out until I could time his next inspiration. Then, the moment he began to take in a breath, I pushed the tube quickly and firmly downward and let him—essentially—inhale it into his trachea.

Immediately he coughed several times and tried to reach up to pull out the tube. The nurse held his arm, and I quickly reminded him that that was supposed to happen and he would feel better very soon. I now could see more fog and moisture forming on the inside of the tube as the air went in and out, and I could feel the air on my cheek as it went by. The respiratory therapist quickly inflated the balloon, attached the ventilation bag, and once more took over the patient's breathing.

Once more it seemed to work. The patient relaxed and immediately ceased fighting the tube, allowing the air to go in and out. I ordered a stat portable chest X-ray to verify that the tube was in the right place, and it came back a few minutes later showing that it was. His oxygen level bumped up a percentage point or two. Once more things seemed to be better. I had his breathing under my control and he could rest a little. All I had to do now was make sure his ventilator settings were correct, that he was oxygenating, and that we were getting out the carbon dioxide, and then send him upstairs.

Or at least that was what I had hoped would happen.

For five or ten minutes, I thought we were out of the woods. He seemed to relax, and his pO_2 stabilized, though this time around 90 or 91. I think I sent a blood sample to the lab to test chemically for the oxygen and carbon dioxide in his blood. I tried thinking about any other possible diagnosis that might be making this happen. Pneumonia? I hadn't seen it on

X-ray, and he hadn't been systemically ill. Blood clot to the lungs? Possible, but that should not have caused such severe wheezing, and in any case in those days there was nothing I could do about it. A reaction to the medicines? It was possible, but I didn't think it was likely. He had been on albuterol for years without problems. And an adverse reaction to steroids would be even more unlikely. The chest X-ray I had just taken showed marked hyperinflation but no other critical abnormality.

I was debating with myself whether to repeat the X-ray when everything fell apart.

Many people have had the experience of driving on an icy road in winter. Everything is under control. You are going slowly, very attentive to the road, looking for ice, not touching the brakes or accelerator any more than you need to, holding the steering wheel gently. Occasionally you have a quick moment of skidding, but you can keep steering in the direction you are going and your wheels catch.

Then, all at once, things break loose. Suddenly you are in a real skid and the wheels aren't catching. Now the car is slowly rotating in a circle. You can see the ditch alongside the road as you slowly head toward it and, at the same time, the headlights of an oncoming car. Time has slowed down. Everything you see is sharp and clear. A part of you can't believe that this is happening: you will get out of this; you will miss the bank; the car will miss you. But the car keeps turning, the other car is coming closer even as you continue to spin toward the side of the road, and you have already done everything you know how to do.

That was how it felt.

First it was his shoulders. Suddenly behind his clavicle on the right side, a large lump formed, and then another. And then it started happening on the left side. I felt them with my fingers and could feel their surface give as if I were pushing on a balloon full of air—which was exactly what it was.

The pictures I have in my memory are blurry; I can't really see his face. But as I write this, I still can see the lumps popping up on his shoulders like a plague of boils, and I can feel the slight crunchy feeling under my fingers, like pressing on the air-filled plastic wrap that comes inside shipping boxes. And even as I watched, I heard the nurse start calling out the slow, steady drop of his pO_2.

It wasn't a pneumothorax. Pneumothorax—literally "air in the chest"—is the name for what happens when an air passage in the lungs springs a leak, and air starts being pushed out into the space between the lung and the chest wall. If it happens under pressure, it is possible to pump so much air out into the chest cavity that the lungs cannot inflate, and the patient will suffocate.

But that's not what he had. It's true that the pressure in his lungs, as he tried to empty them, was too great. Somewhere, probably quite close to the large bronchi, something had indeed popped, and now with each breath, while he continued to pump air out of his lungs, some of it was leaking out into his mediastinum. This is the mass of fibrous tissue between the two lungs, in which the heart and great blood vessels lie. It extends upward from the heart, following the blood vessels and the trachea, and opens out into the bottom of the neck, merging with the connective tissue there. And as the air that was being pumped into it had nowhere else to go, it went upward, dissecting through the tissue and into his neck and shoulders.

Unlike a pneumothorax, the air from the pneumomediastinum caused no breathing problems. However, like a tire with a nail puncture, the respiratory tract had still developed a leak and no longer could maintain pressure. And without that pressure, oxygen was not being driven into the bloodstream anymore.

And there was not a damned thing I could do about it.

But there was one thing I could do: I could suspect that it might be associated with something I could fix. Perhaps the mediastinum was not the only place where the lung was leaking. Perhaps it was leaking also into the chest cavity, between the lung and the chest wall. In that case, the air would not only be leaking out of the lung, it would also start taking up space where the lung should be. And if this continued, the pumping action of his breathing would quickly inflate that space and cause the lung to collapse.

Was it happening? I didn't know; I still don't know. I listened carefully to the lungs on both sides, but they seemed the same, both distant and soft. Were they collapsing? Or was it just that he could no longer move much air? The only way to really tell was to get a chest X-ray—but this man was going to be dead long before that could be done.

But if I couldn't treat a pneumomediastinum, I could goddamn well treat a pneumothorax.

Which was what I did. I grabbed a chest tube tray and

opened it. And I believe I splashed a little Betadine on his chest. I did not use lidocaine; his eyes were closed, and he was making no respiratory efforts to aid the ventilator. He still had a pulse, however, so I went ahead. I took a scalpel and made a stab wound just above the bottom of his fourth or fifth rib on the left side, then slid the blade up to the top of the rib and then almost all the way through into the lung. Then, so as not to damage the lung, I took a blunt clamp and poked a hole into the chest cavity, and then put in a gloved finger. When I did so, I could feel lung firmly against my finger: it was not a large pneumothorax if any at all. But now he had a hole in his chest and I had to finish the procedure. So next, I slid a large chest tube through the hole in his chest while the nurse attached the other end to a water seal so that air could escape but not enter, and I asked the nurse to seal it with tape.

Then I did the same thing on the right side. With the same result.

That was all I could do. By now his oxygen was below 80 percent and dropping quickly. He had not responded in the slightest to what should have been two painful procedures. And his heart rate on the monitor, which had started dropping as I started the procedures, was now below 30, and I could no longer feel a pulse.

And I had run out of things I knew how to do.

The nurses and the respiratory therapist and I stood silent for a few minutes until his last few heartbeats had flitted like fitful hiccups across the screen. I asked them whether they had any thoughts or had questions I could answer. I don't remember if they did. Then I thanked them and went back to the physician's area to write my note.

There is no good end to this story. There are only questions.

Why did he die? The autopsy concluded that it was severe COPD with an acute exacerbation of his underlying asthma and an associated pneumomediastinum. But that doesn't answer the questions of why now; why so bad; why so quickly? I have thought about a paradoxical reaction to albuterol, causing the bronchioles to constrict instead of dilate, and I still think it is possible. However, he had been using the medication for much of his life without problems. More recently I have wondered whether his extremely hyperinflated lungs may have put enough pressure on his mediastinum to decrease blood flow return to the heart. Or maybe he really had a pneumothorax and I just did not reach it with my tubes. I don't know.

The thing I still think most about is, did I make a mistake? Was there something else I could have done at that time that might have made a difference, that even now I have not recognized? I talked it over with my group, and they had no suggestions. And people do die on ordinary days, when they are not expecting to do so.

But I still wonder.

CHAPTER TWENTY

Dead Drunk

N OT EVERY MEMORY is grim. I have one of a disheveled, obviously intoxicated man who just wasn't sobering up fast enough.

The police had brought him in about midnight. He could walk and talk and moved his limbs well. His pupils responded appropriately when I shined a light in them. He knew his name and where he lived. However, he remembered nothing about what he had been doing that evening. And of course, he reeked of alcohol, his speech was slurred, he was generally confused, and he could not walk a straight line.

The police had found him lying passed out on the lawn in front of his house. No one else was home, so they figured he must have just been drinking at home alone and gone outside. It was a warm night, and maybe he wanted to sit on his porch. Then at some point he must have gotten up, wandered out onto the lawn, and passed out. They had thought of just taking him to jail to sober up but decided to take him to the ER to be medically cleared. A lot of people used to come through our ER for similar reasons. They still do.

However, there is nothing about being drunk that protects

you from other problems. So to be on the safe side, I checked his blood sugar. That was normal. Okay, he wasn't a diabetic having an insulin reaction. I also asked the nurse to give him an injection of Narcan. This is a drug that reverses the effects of narcotics—and in doing so detects them. No response to that. Next, because alcoholics frequently have replaced good nutrition for alcohol, and may be dangerously vitamin deficient, I also requested that she give him a shot of thiamine and hang a "banana bag." This was ER jargon for an IV bag containing a salt solution for rehydration and a bunch of water-soluble vitamins. The vitamins color the solution yellow, hence the name. Finally, I ordered a blood alcohol level test and a toxicology screen to check for the presence of other drugs of abuse.

Then, when all the IVs were started and the labs drawn, I ordered the most useful test in all of emergency medicine: I asked that he be put in an observation bed, where he could be evaluated frequently by the nursing staff. Then I went on to the next patient.

It must have been a busy night, because the blood alcohol level took nearly an hour to come back. As I recall, it was moderately high: a little over 0.2 percent or so. That would be enough to put me to sleep, but many heavy drinkers can have a level that high and appear normal.

Around that time, the nurse in charge of the observation unit came up to me looking worried. I asked if he was getting worse. "Well, no," she said. "He's still sleeping comfortably."

"But you are still worried?" I asked.

"Yes," she said. "I mean, he shouldn't be. It's been an hour, and he should be starting to wake up and be hungover. But he isn't."

So I went to see him myself.

She was right; he was sleeping peacefully. As I recall, he had a slight snore. I shook him gently, and in response he lifted his hand and pushed me away. But that was all. He didn't say anything or open his eyes. When I stopped shaking him, he put his arm back down and went back to sleep. I shook him again and called his name. He pushed me away again and this time opened his eyes a little and said something garbled to me. But again, he went right back to sleep. If anything, he was acting a little more drunk than he had been an hour ago.

That's not how it's supposed to work. When you are drunk and go to bed, you sleep it off. Your body consumes the alcohol at a predictable rate. By now he should have been more arousable. And he wasn't.

But what was wrong? He was drinking and had passed out on the lawn of his own front yard. Yes, he was disheveled and smelled of alcohol, but there were no marks on his head or other signs of injury, and there had been nothing at the scene to indicate a source of injury.

Even so.

In the ER, the question is not so much what is likely; it is what are the unlikely but possible things that can hurt you if we miss them. In his case, it was a hidden brain injury, so I sent him to CT.

But then, while I was waiting for the result, the policemen who had found him had called us back. They had made another discovery.

It seems that shortly after they had dropped off our patient, they had been called to an accident about two blocks away. A car going at high speed had crashed into a tree. The odd thing was that there weren't any victims at the scene. The driver's-side door was open and no one was there. So they checked the registration and . . . yep: the name on the card was that of my patient. We finally figured out what must have happened.

He had been drunk. But he had not been drinking at home. He had been drinking at a bar a couple of miles away. Then, while driving home, he had hit the tree. He had most likely been wearing his seat belt, which was why he was relatively uninjured. He was only two blocks from home, so he got out of his car and staggered the rest of the way.

Then he had an incredible stroke of luck: he did not quite make it into the house.

Instead, just before arriving at his front door, he passed out on the lawn for the police to find him. And then, to his equal good fortune, the police decided not to let him sleep it off in jail but to take him to the hospital instead.

Fortunate? How so? Because around that time, the CT scan came back.

It seems that in the crash, even though he had been wearing his seat belt and had not actually struck his head, his brain had been shaken hard enough inside his skull to tear some small veins that run from the skull to the coverings of the brain. Then, slowly over the next couple of hours, he developed a moderately large collection of blood under his skull—which was just starting to press on his brain. However, it was still early in the process, so there was time for the neurosurgeon to drill some holes in his skull and drain the blood.

If he had made it the last few steps into his house and then passed out, he might never have woken up again.

CHAPTER TWENTY-ONE

An Extraordinary Day

O N OUR FIRST day of medical school, the dean of students stood in front of the class, casually spinning his reflex hammer as if it were a six-shooter, and said that half of what they were about to teach us was wrong. The problem was that they didn't know which half. Finding that out was going to be our job.

He was wrong. It turned out to be much more than half. In fact, the one thing in medicine that is certain is that nothing is certain, and most of the surprises are not happy ones.

Most. But not all.

Another summer's day at University Hospital in Augusta, Georgia. The head nurse told me that the paramedic ambulance was bringing in a ten-year-old boy. He had been swimming with his friends in one of the canals that paralleled the nearby Savannah River when he went underwater and did not come back up. One of his friends had run to a phone and called 911. The paramedics arrived promptly and, with the friends' help, managed to find the boy and drag him out of the water. They started CPR immediately and were en route. By the time I got there, they were expected any minute.

The nurses were already setting up for the resuscitation.

University Hospital has the second-busiest ER in the state of Georgia—roughly sixty-five thousand patient visits a year— and we had lots of help. One nurse was assigned to do chest compressions, rotating with the other nurses who were pulling medications into syringes, setting up IVs, and getting the EKG monitor ready. The respiratory therapist was at the head of the bed, ready to manage the child's breathing. The chaplain and patient representative had both been paged.

The canal was not far from the hospital, and in moments the ambulance was there with the boy. The EMTs did their swift dance of movement, transfer, and continued CPR, handing control carefully to the nurses, and then stood back by the wall, at once available to help and out of the way. The paramedic handed me the run sheet. It told the brief story of the rescue: of being called, of getting to the scene, of finding him in the water and assisting in getting him out, beginning CPR at the side of the canal, getting no response, intubating him, and transferring him to the hospital. Two numbers stood out from the rest. The first was the time that the 911 call had been placed; and the second was the time he was finally pulled from the water.

The difference between them was fifteen minutes.

"Are these good numbers? He was under for fifteen minutes?" I asked. The paramedic nodded.

I remember looking at the boy. He looked his age—healthy and strong, just beginning the adolescent growth spurt that would take him to his dangerous teenage years, and then to manhood. But like the little girl years before, he too was limp, unresponsive, making no attempt to breathe, pupils wide.

And of course, the tracing of his heart rhythm on the monitor was a straight flat line.

In short, he was dead.

Right about then, a prematurely silver-haired, heavy-set man casually wandered through the doorway of the resuscitation room. He was calm, and quiet, as if he were confident that everything in the world was going just fine. If the trauma room had been a kitchen, and he was just seeing whether we needed help with the dishes, he could not have been more relaxed and matter-of-fact. His name was Dick Eckert. He was the other emergency physician/pediatrician in our group.

I don't remember whether he was working clinically that day or had just stopped by to do some paperwork. It doesn't matter. He had a way of showing up at moments when no one else would do.

"Need any help?" he asked.

"Absolutely," I said. "Ten years old. Documented underwater at least fifteen minutes before they pulled him out."

Dick nodded. Then we both looked at the cardiac rhythm visible on the monitor. "Looks like fine V-fib to me," I said. "What do you think?"

He glanced at me and nodded. "Could be," he said. And so we—Dick and I, and the nurses and the respiratory therapist—all began a battle against death that we knew we had no hope of winning.

In my memory, I have always divided the next hour into three parts: Here We Go Again; Oh My God; and What Have We Done?

You already know about Here We Go Again: continue CPR; check the tube; check pulses; check the tracing. Then shock, shock, shock and so on down the line. In my memory, Dick was everywhere: helping me make sure I wasn't screwing up on any of the drugs or voltages, as well as being a peer who kept me company in a clinically and emotionally difficult situation. He was also alternating with the nurses on chest compressions and helping the respiratory therapist manage the tube in the boy's windpipe. Also, because he was there, after about ten minutes I could leave the resuscitation and go out to the family room, where the mother was sitting with other family members, and tell her how things were going.

I was not optimistic. I felt that my job was to help her with her expectations so that when, in a few minutes, I would most certainly have to go in to tell her that her son was dead, the news would not be completely unexpected, and that the family and friends with her would be prepared to help her. I spoke to her for a few minutes, then went back to the resuscitation.

It seems to me that by that time they were somewhere around the second dose of lidocaine. As a procedure, the resuscitation was going smoothly. The boy was being well ventilated with oxygen via the endotracheal tube; people were trading off on chest compression at regular intervals; the bretylium was given precisely on time and then followed by another shock.

The only problem was that there was no sign that we were accomplishing anything. The tracing on the monitor showed absolutely no change from a flat straight line. As confirmation, the boy still had no pulse. At that point, there was nothing left for us to do, so Dick and I looked at each other and got ready to quit.

Which was when Oh My God started.

Suddenly, on the monitor there was a quick upright wave, an electrical impulse consistent with a heartbeat. That didn't mean that the boy had really been in fine ventricular fibrillation and we had just succeeded in shocking him out of it. That would have led to a regular succession of impulses. But there was just one, which smoothly slid off the screen as the tracing progressed. We waited, but nothing further happened.

I turned to Dick. "That's just a terminal rhythm, isn't it?" By that I meant the occasional random contraction of an essentially dead heart. I don't remember a reply; Dick never said more than he had to. Now he just watched the screen.

And suddenly there was another.

"Did he have a pulse with that?" I asked. The nurse shook his head.

"Well, let's keep on going," I said.

Which was just what we did—for another twenty minutes, watching as the number of impulses on the screen gradually increased, until they were occurring eighty or ninety times a minute—approximately a normal rate. And then, the nurse said, "I think I feel a pulse."

Which was when What Have We Done? started to happen.

Because it was clear by then that, by some unexplainable chance, we had first gotten his heart restarted, and then it was sufficiently undamaged to have a regular beat, and finally it was strong enough to pump blood through his body. Unfortunately, however, it was not only his heart that had been starved for oxygen. His brain had been as well. And brains are far more easily damaged by a lack of blood flow than hearts.

In an earlier part of my career, when I was still a practicing pediatrician, I had served as a consultant to the North Coast Regional Center (now the Redwood Coast Regional Center) office in Ukiah. This was—and is—the organization that provides services to neurologically handicapped children and adults. Among our clients were two or three patients who, as children, had drowned, had been without oxygen for a prolonged period, and then had been resuscitated. Without exception, their deficits were profound. Unable to talk, walk, or even feed themselves, unable even to truly demonstrate their ability to think, these patients lived because their parents spent most of their waking hours, and much of their lives, caring for them. We were resuscitating a child who had been under warm water for at least fifteen minutes, if not longer, and whose heart had stopped for over half an hour. Were we saving a life that would be worth living?

Almost at once, we had evidence that we were not: the boy started having seizures. He had at least three or four over the next twenty minutes. His body tensed, his extremities jerked, his teeth clenched around the ET tube—each seizure lasted a minute or so, after which he lapsed once more into limp unresponsiveness.

We gave him antiseizure medications intravenously— lorazepam and then phenobarbital—and finally, the seizures stopped. But the boy remained unconscious and unarousable.

Then, right after the last dose of anticonvulsant medication, the pediatric intensive care staff arrived to take him upstairs. At this point, an hour had passed since he had come in the door.

I thanked the nursing staff for their help. They had been the ones who had done the care that we directed, and it was the quality of their work as much or more than ours that had brought him back. Dick smiled at me, said "Nice job," and left. I went to talk to the mother one last time.

I told her that, almost unbelievably, her child was alive and was heading up to the ICU. At the same time I had to tell her that he might not be the same child; that he could likely have had significant brain injury, and that he had almost certainly swallowed water, so that the chance of a lung infection was very real. In short, the job was just beginning.

She shook my hand, thanked me, and went to see her son, and I went back to work in the pediatric emergency department. What I did there the rest of that day, I cannot even begin to recall.

But I remember very clearly coming to work the next morning. Before going on shift, I went upstairs to the pediatric ICU, walked up to the main desk, and asked what bed the boy was in. The nurse looked at me and pointed to a room just behind her. "That was his room . . . but he's gone."

I nodded sadly. "What time did he die?" I asked.

"You don't understand," she said. "He's gone. He was discharged. He went home."

"He went home?" I said. I must have sounded as if I were deaf.

"Yes," she said. "He woke up about midnight and was fine.

Walking, talking, eating, no signs of pneumonia. Mom was there so they sent him home with her."

I shook my head and then, still not really believing it, I went down to tell the ER staff that they had had a save.

I did get one other bit of follow-up. A week or so later I was working with Glenn Bridges, one of the other emergency physicians, and he said something to the effect of did I remember that boy last week who drowned? I braced myself for the bad news and asked what happened. I was sure he was going to tell me how the boy had come back to the ER with terrible seizures or some other evidence of permanent brain damage.

What he said was, "Well, he came in yesterday afternoon with a laceration on his hand. He and his friends were climbing a fence, and he cut himself on the wire." Glenn smiled at me. "He was fine," he said.

Epilogue

ONE OF THE problems with being a physician is that usually you must wait until the end of your career to taste the bread you bake. Most of us begin our medical education in our twenties. That's an age at which most people think that being sick means that you have the flu, and that all medication prescriptions end with the words "for ten days." I was no exception. In addition, by good fortune, I can only remember three occasions in my life when I had to go to the hospital for an emergency.

The first time was when I was five. My parents and I were at a seafood restaurant, and I got a bone stuck in my throat. All I remember of the ER is being in the waiting room for what seemed a long time, and then lying on my back, looking up at the doctor. He had a light on his forehead and a couple of scary instruments in each hand. Fortunately, as I waited for him to do whatever he was going to do, I suddenly swallowed the bone.

The next time was when I was nine. My parents took me to the hospital at night because of a fever and a lot of muscle aches. The doctor thought I might have polio, so he put me in the hospital, where twice a day for two weeks, a nurse shot penicillin into my butt. Then they decided I didn't have polio after all and let me go back to school. The penicillin did me no good. Polio is a virus, and antibiotics have no effect on viruses. But this was 1952, and nobody knew that.

The last time was when I was twelve. I was attending a school in the Adirondack Mountains, and in the winter we could ski. There were no such things as safety releases in those days. One day I fell, twisting my foot and ankle, so a teacher had to take me to the hospital in Lake Placid. The doctor examined the injury, took an X-ray, and decided it was only a sprain.

So three ER visits, and each time I escaped intact. And for the next sixty years, that was that. I don't mean that I have never been ill. Ever since I finished my residency, I have always had a physician for my annual physicals and ongoing health care. It's just that, since childhood, I have never needed to go to the emergency room.

Until a year ago.

My wife and I own a small RV. Really, it's just a Dodge cargo van that has acquired a very serious case of Winnebago. So far the disease has replaced much of its cargo-carrying equipment with beds and sinks and stoves and the like, and the end is not in sight. One spring afternoon I was cleaning it out to get ready for a trip south when I slipped and fell. On the way to the floor, I struck my left hip on the pointed corner of the wooden bed frame.

The pain was like nothing I had ever before experienced. In addition, just like in the TV commercial, I really had fallen and could not get up. Fortunately, I had my phone in my pocket, so I called my wife, who was at her desk in the house, and asked if she might come out to the van and either shoot me or help me try to stand. She came at once and, to my good fortune, chose the second alternative. Getting me off the floor was a challenge, but between her grunts and my groans, I ultimately found myself upright.

At that point, I discovered that I could not bear weight on my left leg. Even moving it made the pain worse. So despite my nearly infinite capacity for denial, I had to ask myself whether I might not have broken my hip. And of course, there was only one way to find out: I had to go to the emergency room.

The next problem was getting me there. I don't really remember how she did it. I am almost six feet tall and, on a light day, weigh 175 pounds. Linda, on the other hand, is gradually drifting below five feet two. Even so, she somehow maneuvered me, at a half hop, half drag, into our actual car and drove me to the nearest hospital, all the while being forced to listen to me whine and moan every time she used the brakes or hit a bump. But even in the midst of my discomfort, I realized that something new and important was happening to me: for the first time since I was that twelve-year-old boy with a sore ankle, I was being "rushed to the emergency room." (Slowly and carefully rushed. At the speed limit, all the way.) I was enormously curious what it would be like.

When we arrived, Linda pulled up to the ambulance entrance and went inside. Seconds later she was back with two nurses and a wheelchair. They asked if I could walk. I said not bloody likely. Then they asked if they could help me into the wheelchair. The ride over had not caused too much additional pain, and I knew I wasn't getting into the ER until I got out of the car, so I agreed. So "gently but firmly," that's exactly what they did. It hurt, of course, but no more than it had to. Then they took me to a room and with equal care loaded me onto a gurney.

When I was settled, one of the nurses started asking me the basic historical questions. How old was I? Seventy-two. Was I allergic to any medications? No. Did I have any significant illnesses or prior hospitalizations? A few. And so on. He was rapid but thorough and missed nothing of importance. After he finished, the ward clerk came in, asked my name and address and a few other identifiers, and then borrowed my insurance cards to copy. That took maybe a minute. Obviously, none of this was surprising. I have been a part of this routine for much of my life. But while it was completely the same, it was also utterly different. It was as if I were in the same room in which I had always worked, but standing on the ceiling instead of on the floor. Everything was familiar, but it was all upside down. Suddenly I was on the receiving end. This time I was the customer in a restaurant where I had spent my life waiting on tables.

Then a small miracle happened. Only a minute or two later, the other nurse came back holding two small syringes. He asked me to hold out my arm, and then he slipped a small IV line into a vein in the back of my hand. As he did so, he asked me to rate my pain from one to ten. By that point, it had come down from a nine to about a six. So he asked me if I would like some medication for the pain.

I hesitated for a moment. The pain was a bit better, and I didn't want to seem like a wimp. Also—well, there is an epidemic of opioid addiction going on in this country, and I didn't want them to think I was just there for drugs. So I said maybe I could hold off for now.

But then he said something that was both thoughtful and important: "Remember, in a little while you are going to go to the X-ray department; they will move you onto a table, and once you are there, they will have to move your hip around a bit. That will probably hurt a lot. Are you sure you don't want something?"

He was right. That was exactly what was going to happen. I nodded and held out my arm.

The medication they gave me was not strong. Its principal component is similar to what's in Aleve, though a little stronger and able to be given as a shot. Even so, quickly my pain went down to a very manageable three.

Soon after that the physician's assistant came in. He also took a brief history and in addition did a gentle examination, both palpating and manipulating my hip. It hurt a bit—but was bearable. When he finished, he said that he doubted I had broken my hip, but that's what the X-ray machine was for. Then he asked if I had any questions—I didn't—and said he would talk to me again when I was back from the radiology department.

The radiology techs were quick and careful. They too understood the issue of pain. Yes, they had to move my hip around a little, and yes, it hurt, but not very much—especially with the medication on board. And then they rolled me back to the ER.

The PA had been correct. Not too long after I returned from radiology, he came back into the room and told me that indeed it was not broken. It was just badly bruised over the joint so that in addition to the pain of the injury, moving the leg aggravated the pain. Then—though he had known from the beginning of my visit that I was an emergency physician who had given the same instructions thousands of times myself—he went over the medication he was sending me home with, the likely duration of my symptoms, and a review of the written instructions provided by the computer. He closed with an invitation to return anytime if things did not go well. He did not insult my intelligence when he did so; he simply took nothing for granted, and I was grateful he did not. Then he gave me some papers to sign and a sheaf of discharge instructions for me to review at my leisure. All that was left was another wheelchair ride to our car, and I was on my way home, feeling better. The whole visit took maybe an hour. And once more I had gotten in and out of the ER without any terrible discoveries. I was lucky of course. They weren't very busy, and my injury was not complex.

More important, the ER to which I had gone was staffed with excellent people, who worked in a hospital that strives to have a culture of caring—something that all hospitals try to do, of course, with varying success. Oddly enough, the fact that I was "one of them" didn't make much of a difference. They knew what I had done for a living, but they never assumed anything because of that, and always treated me like a patient, not a peer.

My ER visit was fortunate, but it was also revealing: in a way I had never before experienced, I had a feeling for what mattered to me about my visit. And I think it is possible that other people might have some similar feelings.

First, it mattered to me how I was welcomed. Few people come to the ER just because they are bored and want some entertainment. Most of the time, whatever their problem is, they feel it to be both important and one that only an emergency room can solve. It matters if the people who greet you on your arrival seem to understand that and seem to care.

Second, it mattered how I was initially evaluated. Most people know that patients are triaged—prioritized in terms of need—and that more minor problems may need to wait. But they do want to be prioritized correctly—to know that the treatment for their pain or their fear is not being inappropriately delayed because of someone else's less critical problem. Furthermore, if they do have to wait, they want to know from time to time that they are not forgotten, even if it's only a brief word. Third, it mattered to me that the people treating me appeared both competent and caring.

It is true that actual competence is something that most people cannot judge. They assume that the hospital has made sure that the people caring for them are competent, just as we all assume that airlines ensure that their pilots are competent. But they certainly can, and will, judge how much the staff seems to care—and whether they seem competent in the process.

Finally, it mattered to me that when I left the hospital, I felt that I had received the service I had wanted. That should be obvious, but it does not always occur. Just as at a restaurant you expect a good meal, and are annoyed when the food is bad, patients want to feel that they have received the help they came for.

That help may take many forms. It may be a prescription, a procedure, or an appropriate referral or transfer. It may be as serious as an admission to the hospital, or as minor as a set of instructions that have been reviewed and explained by the person who took care of them. Or, most important, it may be the reassurance that the thing they feared is not what is actually happening to them: that they are not having a stroke or a heart attack or whatever. In short, as in any other business, they have purchased a product and they want to be able to take it home. As I said, I was fortunate; the service I needed was exactly the service I received.

But I know also that not all visits are like that. While I feel that people who work in emergency rooms are among the finest people I have known, I also know that ERs are often overcrowded, and sometimes short-staffed. I have worked in ERs in which those situations were so common that chart racks were installed in the hallways, in order to identify places to park patients when all the rooms were full. And everyone knows that the service the ER provides is not cheap. However, none of these issues represent the wishes of those who work in the ER. They are instead the direct result of our national ambivalence over health care: we want the best, but we are unwilling to pay for it.

From time to time over the years, I have been asked how long I think it will take before the American health care system collapses. My answer has always been the same: "It has already collapsed; it did so years ago. But because of the emergency rooms in our country, we have not yet had to face that fact." To put this another way, a family has been defined as the group that has to take you in when no one else will. However, when your nation, your government, and even your family have all abandoned you, you can still come to the emergency room.

Let me close with one more brief story.

Some years ago, I was at an educational meeting where I listened to a talk given by an emergency physician on the subject of interacting with patients. Recently he had taken care of a small child with meningitis. Everyone had done their jobs well. The patient had been rapidly assessed, quickly treated with the appropriate antibiotics, and ultimately survived intact. After all the work was finished, and the patient was waiting to go up to the pediatric intensive care unit, the doctor sat and talked with the child's mother, asking how she was doing, and whether she had any questions. She said no. But then she thanked him and told him how frightened she had been on the way to the hospital.

"Because of not knowing what was wrong with your child?" he asked.

"No," she said. "I knew that he was very sick. I was terrified because I didn't know who you would be."

I have been lucky. Even so, I know that somewhere up ahead, there awaits an ER visit that will not be so benign. However, I am confident that when that happens, even if I have never met them before, I will be among competent and caring friends. As, I believe, will you.

Acknowledgments

First, I thank my friends, simply for being my friends. I won't name anyone: you all know who you are, in what way you are my friend, and how grateful I am for having had you in my life. If I were to use names, then some would be missed, and that would defeat the message I want to send: You and my family are the foundation of my life, that which supports me in everything I do, and I am forever grateful.

However, regarding the book, specific thanks are needed. I must begin with Sharon Carmack. She teaches an online course in writing nonfiction for Southern New Hampshire University that I took a few years ago. (The chapter "Shears" began as an assignment for her course.) She taught me a lot about writing, but most of all I learned from her to trust that writing was something I could do.

There are also three people who, in addition to being friends, did me the extra favor of not only reading the entire book but also of telling me in detail what they thought worked and what didn't, and by the way, you forgot a comma on page 129. Two of them were Mike and Lucy Harrison, each of whom reviewed it individually, even though they have been hanging out together for well over a half century and could have done it as a committee. Tom Jackson also critiqued it, but in addition, he casually mentioned that in a previous life he had been a manager of a publishing company. Accordingly, so I wouldn't be too annoyed or terrified if by some chance it happened, he walked me through the intricate task of taking a bunch of marks on a computer screen and making them into a Real Live Book.

Which leads me to Catapult. Everyone at Catapult has been wonderful. But some people I must mention in particular.

Megha Majumdar has been my Guide in Chief through all the bits and pieces Tom warned me about. She has used, as needed, a laser, a scalpel, and a battle-ax on my choicest prose and—to my amazement—made it better. Furthermore, whenever I whined and held my breath about some change or another, she was the soul of patience. In fact, she even let me win a few times. Who could ask for more?

Next, like a drill sergeant at a barracks inspection, Jane Elias ran her white-gloved hands all over what I thought were spotless pages, and brought them back filthy with misplaced commas, random capitalizations, grammatical disasters, and the like. But unlike a sergeant, she has had only the gentlest of requests and the kindest of remonstrations.

Last but not least, as the publication date continues to approach, I have also come to appreciate the work of the people who are the business end of the book business, the real reason that you—or someone you know, who likes you enough to lend you things—actually bought this book. These include Erin Kottke, and Jenn Abel Kovitz, who let you know that you might enjoy reading it; and finally Wah-Ming Chang, managing editor, the person at the end of this whole process who made sure that the book said what it was supposed to say, precisely as it was meant to say it.

So Ms. Strachan, for all this and more, next time coffee is on me.

But I would never have found Megha, or Catapult, without Wendy Levinson of the Harvey Klinger Agency. My records indicate that she was the twenty-sixth agent to whom I submitted my manuscript. However, rough as it was, she actually read it, liked it, and, most astonishing, understood what I was trying to say. Having done so, she made me trash enough irrelevant material that a publisher might feel the same way. Now, virtually daily, she guides me through the perils of the Book Business. (Also, she was on her college ski team and still likes skiing the bumps. I am totally awestruck.)

But before all of them, there was my family. As with my friends, that is a circle whose boundaries are blurry. Even so, some people need special mention. My mother, father, and stepfather: you departed long ago for even more fascinating conversations elsewhere, but I thank you anyway for everything you gave me; perhaps you are listening. My brother, Bowen: thank you for your encouragement and for being my brother when being a stepbrother was all that was in the job description. My nephew, Jim, and the whole Ehlen-Hren household: thank you all for creating a place that, every time I enter, feels like I've come home. Cousin Nikki: thank you for regularly stopping by to bring your brand of happiness into our lives. My son, Nick: thank you for your enthusiasm—and for not giving up.

Finally, Linda . . .

Linda, of course I thank you for reading the book. I thank you for telling me it was good where it was good and bad where it was bad. But that is small potatoes compared to the task of putting up with me for nearly fifty years. I love thee with the breath, smiles, tears of all my life—as well as those other things Ms. Browning mentioned. I cannot imagine spending all those years without you.

Notes

28 "in later years such a schedule would not even be legal": In 1984, an eighteen-year-old girl named Libby Zion died in a New York hospital. Her parents sued, alleging that her death was caused by fatigue on the part of an overworked intern and resident. In 1989 New York State passed the "Libby Zion law," which limited the working hours of house staff to a mere eighty hours per week and no more than twenty-four hours at a single stretch. In 2003 these regulations became the rule nationwide.

32 "blood oxygen saturation": The percentage of oxygen being carried by the red blood cells, compared to their total capacity to carry oxygen. The red cells of a normal person breathing room air at sea level should be completely full of oxygen. However, people with long-term breathing problems often live normally and feel all right with saturations considerably lower.

32 "transposition of the great vessels": Transposition of the great vessels is a condition in which the aorta, the pathway for blood to leave the heart and go throughout the body, is switched with the pulmonary artery, the pathway for blood to go from the heart to the lungs. Normally the circulation of the heart is like a figure skater making a figure eight: blood comes from the body to the right side of the heart via the upper and lower vena cava (Latin for "great vein"). The right ventricle then pumps the blood into the lungs. From there it goes into the left side of the heart via the pulmonary arteries and is pumped from there by the left ventricle into the body again, and the path repeats itself—all in

just about one minute. However, if the aorta and the pulmonary artery happen to be switched, instead of a figure eight, you just have two independent circles of blood that never touch—one going back and forth from the heart to the lungs and the other from the heart to the body. In intrauterine life, this isn't a problem; oxygen for the body isn't coming from the lungs, it's coming from the mother via the placental arteries directly into the body's circulation. Also, did I say never touch? That's not quite true. In neonatal life, there is a connection between the pulmonary artery and the aorta called the ductus arteriosus, which allows some of the blood from the body also to visit the lungs. As long as this is open, the baby has some chance at getting enough oxygen to live. The problem is that within a few days after birth, it will close and the baby will die. This problem is what the resident's baby had.

49 "I wish I knew how it turned out": When this manuscript was finished, I sent it to Drs. Gregory, Phibbs, and Kitterman for their review and comments. In his reply, Dr. Kitterman told me that this child in fact survived her hospitalization, and was followed in their clinic for the next five years, doing well. The thumb that Dr. de Lorimier reattached was smaller than the other, but perfectly functional.

57 "I remember her well": I could not forget her. Though I didn't know it at the time, she was a member of the Peoples Temple, Jim Jones's religious cult, which in those years was located just outside Ukiah, but was soon to relocate to Guyana. I discovered that she was a member only when I found her name (as well as many other names I knew) on the list of people who died there, in the mass murder that Jim Jones directed.

85 "the EKG machine": An EKG measures the path through the heart that the electrochemical signal takes as it triggers a contraction. When some part of the heart is deprived of blood, either temporarily as in angina, or permanently as in a heart attack, the current will no longer be able to go through that spot and must go around it. That will show up on the cardiogram as an abnormal wave tracing. From the location and shape of the tracing, we

can determine approximately where in the heart the damage is happening.

91 "drive at a dangerous speed": The phrase "They rushed him to the emergency room" is one I despise: it implies that something is good and necessary that is in fact always hazardous and almost never helpful. Driving recklessly to get to an emergency room a few moments faster is almost always more dangerous to the patient—and of course to the driver, other passengers, and other vehicles—than driving safely at a normal speed. Most emergency physicians, during their career, have seen family members and friends of patients hurt or killed while "rushing to the emergency room" for problems that were far less important than the damage caused by the driving. Leave rapid transport to the EMTs. They are trained as to when and how to do it, they have flashing lights, sirens, and big vehicles—and even then, every year or so, some of them also are injured and killed while "rushing" patients to the hospital.

93 "So I relax": *Don't* try this at home. At the time of this event, I had been caring for children for approximately twenty years and had indeed seen this—and many other elbow injuries—many times. Elbow injuries are not uncommon, and by no means are all of them nursemaid's elbow.

122 "they really had no idea": That "they really had no idea" is true not only of nonmedical people; doctors and nurses do the same thing. Terrible events are hard for anyone to accept. When one of my nieces developed a hole in a bone in her neck, I managed to convince myself right up to the moment of the surgical biopsy that it must be a low-grade bone infection—instead of the metastasis from a previously undiscovered breast cancer that in any other patient I would have recognized immediately that it was. In the same way, I left my father's bedside in the ICU to go to a business meeting in another state, because I could not let myself realize how close he was to death.

I have not forgotten these—and other—lapses; no one does.

152 "a new onset of angina": "Angina" is short for angina pectoris. This term is from the Latin, meaning "strangulation of the

chest." It is part of the medical spectrum of what is called acute coronary syndrome. Angina, an early stage of acute coronary syndrome, occurs when one of the coronary arteries (the arteries that feed the heart) abruptly becomes sufficiently blocked to deprive the heart muscle of some oxygen but not enough to kill it. The pain of angina is simply because a muscle without oxygen hurts. A myocardial infarction means that the blockage is severe enough that some part of the heart muscle is dying or has died.

Though they are not identical conditions, they are considered part of a spectrum because an artery that is partially closed is perfectly capable of closing completely at any time, changing a new-onset angina attack into a full-fledged myocardial infarction.

152 "blood tests": The blood tests determine whether there are any chemicals running around the bloodstream that normally are found only in the heart. If there are, that means that the heart is leaking juice—and that means there is damage to heart muscle. A positive test is strong evidence of a myocardial infarction. However, a negative test only says that whatever is going on hasn't yet caused enough damage to hurt the heart—but it doesn't say that there is nothing going on. To determine that, we generally need to wait several hours, repeat the tests, and then put the patient on a treadmill to see whether exercise can bring out the problem. Or sometimes, if the history is good enough, the cardiologists just take them to the cardiac catheterization lab to make sure.

209 "physician's assistant": Physician's assistants have two years of academic training compared to the four years that physicians have, and they work under the supervision of a physician. Many rural hospitals are staffed with a single physician medical director who does some clinical work and supervises PAs who work the rest of the shifts as the front-line providers. I have worked for years with PAs in this role, and I include many of them as among the best emergency medicine providers I have had the privilege to know.

And I have to mention that our son is a PA practicing in North-western Virginia.

213 "one more brief story": I do not recall who gave the talk, or I would have given him credit. Let me know who you are; if this book ever has a second edition, you will be in it.